AVOCADO
RECIPES
APPETIZERS, MEALS, SNACKS AND MORE!

Publications International, Ltd.

Pictured on the front cover (*clockwise from top left*): Classic California Burgers (*page 80*), Summer's Best Gazpacho (*page 52*), Go Green Smoothie (*page 11*) and Southwestern Flatbread with Black Beans and Corn (*page 98*).

Pictured on the back cover (*top to bottom*): Pork Tenderloin with Avocado-Tomatillo Salsa (*page 78*), Avocado Lime Pops (*page 113*), and Grilled Chicken with Corn and Black Bean Salsa (*page 90*).

Photography on page 3 © Shutterstock.com

ISBN-13: 978-1-68022-236-4

Library of Congress Control Number: 2015950175

Manufactured in China.

8 7 6 5 4 3 2 1

Microwave Cooking: Microwave ovens vary in wattage. Use the cooking times as guidelines and check for doneness before adding more time.

Preparation/Cooking Times: Preparation times are based on the approximate amount of time required to assemble the recipe before cooking, baking, chilling or serving. These times include preparation steps such as measuring, chopping and mixing. The fact that some preparations and cooking can be done simultaneously is taken into account. Preparation of optional ingredients and serving suggestions is not included.

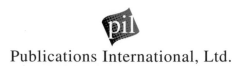

Publications International, Ltd.

TABLE OF CONTENTS

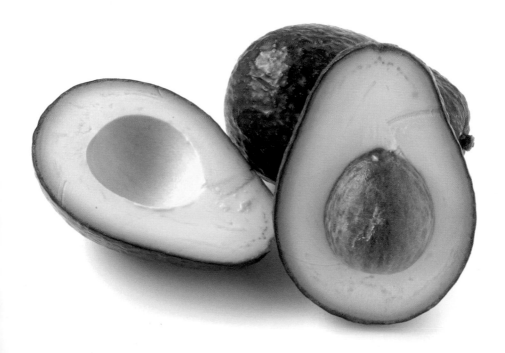

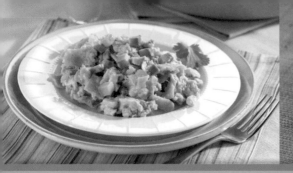
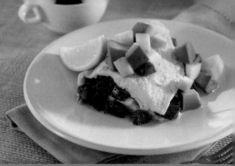

BREAKFAST & BRUNCHES

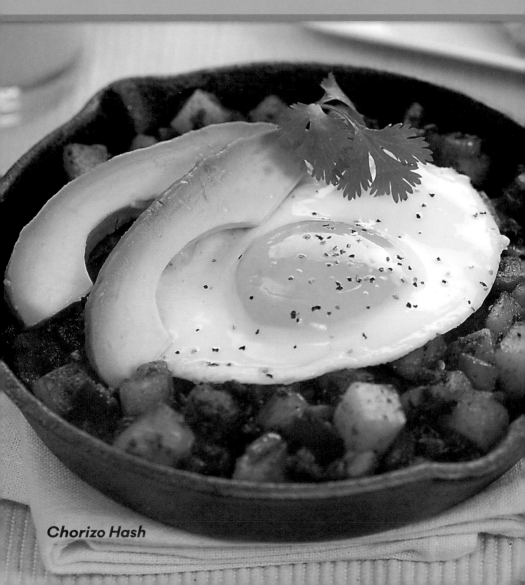

Chorizo Hash

CHORIZO HASH

2 unpeeled russet potatoes, cut into ½-inch pieces

1 tablespoon salt, divided

8 ounces chorizo sausage

1 yellow onion, chopped

½ red bell pepper, chopped (about ½ cup)

Chopped fresh cilantro (optional)

Avocado slices (optional)

1. Fill medium saucepan half full with water. Add potatoes and 2 teaspoons salt; bring to a boil over high heat. Reduce heat to medium-low; cook about 8 minutes. (Potatoes will be firm.) Drain.

2. Meanwhile, remove and discard casing from chorizo. Crumble chorizo into large (12-inch) cast iron skillet; cook and stir over medium-high heat about 5 minutes or until lightly browned. Add onion and bell pepper; cook and stir about 4 minutes or until vegetables are softened.

3. Stir in potatoes and remaining 1 teaspoon salt; cook 10 to 15 minutes or until vegetables are tender and potatoes are lightly browned, stirring occasionally. Garnish with cilantro and avocado.

SERVING SUGGESTION: Serve with fried, poached or scrambled eggs.

BREAKFAST MIGAS

1 **tablespoon olive oil**

1 **small onion, chopped**

1 **jalapeño pepper,* seeded and diced**

3 **corn tortillas, cut into 1-inch pieces**

1 **medium tomato, halved, seeded and diced**

6 **eggs**

2 **tablespoons chunky salsa**

1 **cup (4 ounces) shredded Monterey Jack cheese**

1 **small ripe avocado, diced**

1 **tablespoon lime juice**

Sour cream

Chopped fresh cilantro

*Jalapeño peppers can sting and irritate the skin, so wear rubber gloves when handling peppers and do not touch your eyes.

1. Heat oil in 12-inch nonstick skillet over medium heat. Add onion and jalapeño pepper; cook and stir 1 minute or until soft.

2. Add tortillas and tomato; cook about 2 minutes or until soft and heated through.

3. Slightly beat eggs and salsa in small bowl. Pour mixture into skillet. Cook, stirring occasionally, until eggs are firmly scrambled.

4. Remove skillet from heat; stir in cheese. Garnish each serving with avocado tossed in lime juice, sour cream and cilantro.

NOTE: Migas, a Mexican breakfast dish, is traditionally made in a skillet with leftover, stale tortillas that are torn by hand into small pieces.

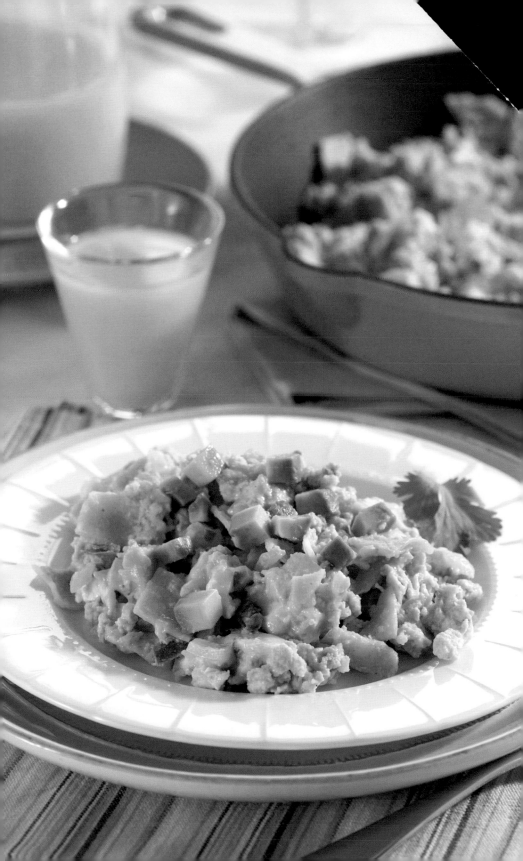

MAKES 2 SERVINGS

2 corn tortillas
1 tomato, diced
1 avocado, diced
¼ teaspoon salt
¼ teaspoon black pepper

¼ teaspoon ground cumin
   Pinch ground red pepper
2 teaspoons olive oil
2 eggs

1. Cut round hole in center of tortillas using 3-inch cookie cutter. Combine tomato, avocado, salt, black pepper, cumin and ground red pepper in small bowl.

2. Heat griddle or large skillet over medium-low heat; brush with oil. Place tortillas in skillet and break 1 egg into center of each hole. Cook 2 to 3 minutes or until whites have firmed. Carefully flip tortilla and egg and cook to desired doneness. Add cut out tortilla rounds to griddle to warm.

3. Serve tortillas and eggs with tomato avocado mixture and top with tortilla round "hats."

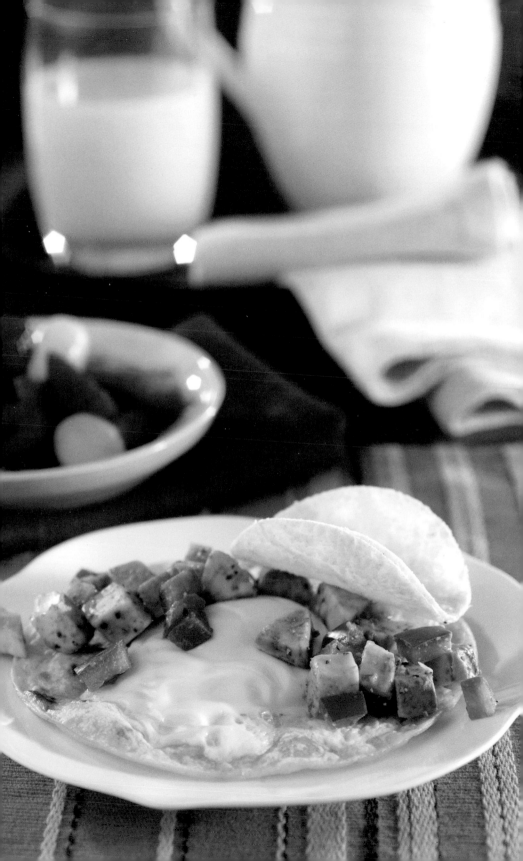

BLUEBERRY CHERRY BLEND

MAKES 2 SERVINGS

¾ **cup water**

¾ **cup frozen blueberries**

¾ **cup frozen dark sweet cherries**

½ **avocado**

1 **tablespoon lemon juice**

1 **teaspoon ground flaxseed**

Combine water, blueberries, cherries, avocado, lemon juice and flaxseed in blender; blend until smooth. Serve immediately.

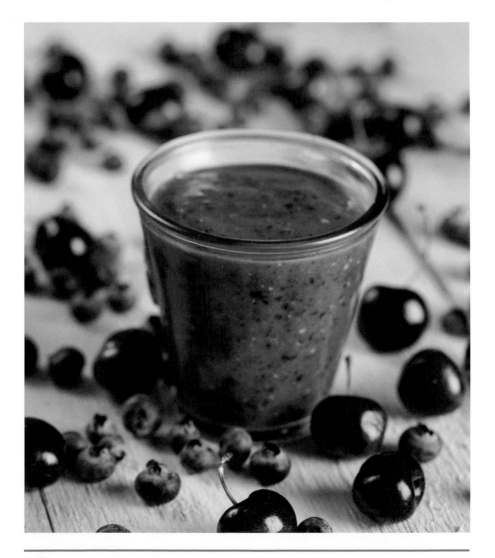

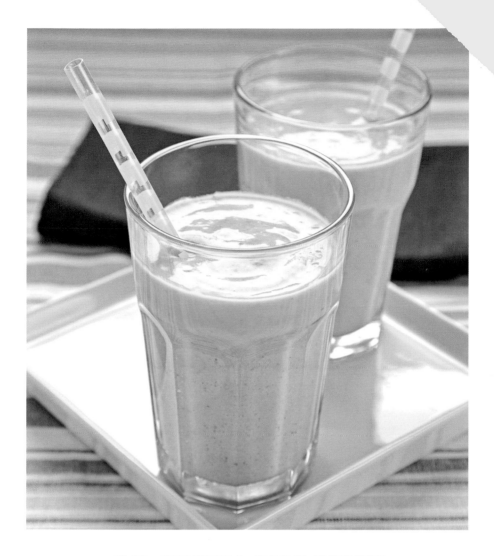

GO GREEN SMOOTHIE

MAKES 1 SERVING

1½ **cups ice cubes**
1 **cup packed torn spinach**
½ **cup vanilla almond milk**
¼ **cup vanilla low-fat yogurt**

¼ **avocado**
1 **teaspoon lemon juice**
1 **teaspoon honey**

Combine ice, spinach, almond milk, yogurt, avocado, lemon juice and honey in blender; blend until smooth.

CALIFORNIA OMELET WITH AVOCADO

MAKES 4 SERVINGS

6 ounces plum tomato, chopped (about 1½ tomatoes)

2 to 4 tablespoons chopped fresh cilantro

¼ teaspoon salt

2 cups cholesterol-free egg substitute

¼ cup fat-free (skim) milk

1 ripe medium avocado, diced

1 small cucumber, chopped

1 lemon, quartered

1. Preheat oven to 200°F. Combine tomatoes, cilantro and salt in small bowl; set aside.

2. Whisk egg substitute and milk in medium bowl until well blended.

3. Heat small nonstick skillet over medium heat; spray with nonstick cooking spray. Pour half of egg mixture into skillet; cook 2 minutes or until eggs begin to set. Lift edge of omelet to allow uncooked portion to flow underneath. Cook 3 minutes or until set.

4. Spoon half of tomato mixture over half of omelet. Loosen omelet with spatula and fold in half. Slide omelet onto serving plate and keep warm in oven. Repeat steps for second omelet with remaining half of egg mixture. Serve topped with avocado and cucumber; garnish with lemon wedges.

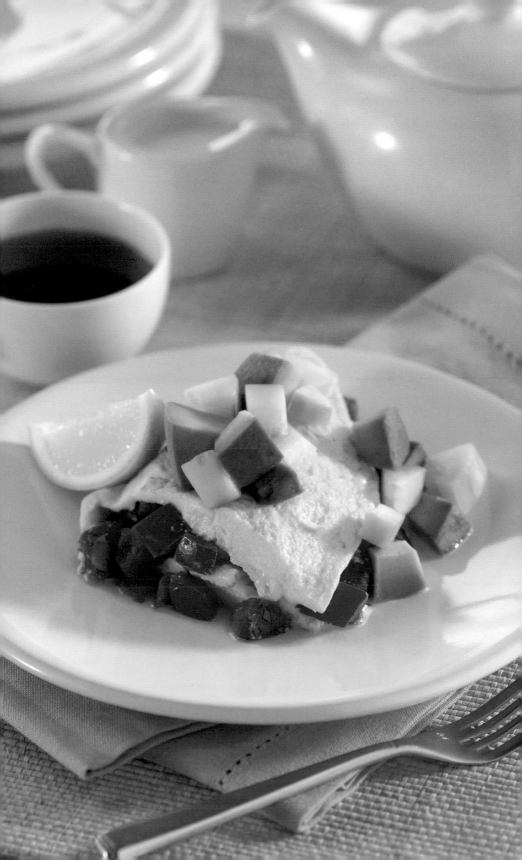

SIESTA RAMEN STRATA

3 packages (3 ounces each) ramen noodles, any flavor*

2 cups (8 ounces) shredded Cheddar cheese

10 large eggs, lightly beaten

4 cups milk

¼ cup chopped red bell pepper

2 tablespoons diced green onions

1 tablespoon chopped fresh cilantro

1 teaspoon salt

⅛ teaspoon ground red pepper

Sour cream, avocado or salsa (optional)

Discard seasoning packets.

1. Spray 13×9-inch baking pan with nonstick cooking spray. Split each noodle square horizontally in two; line pan with noodle squares. Sprinkle cheese over noodles.

2. Whisk eggs, milk, bell pepper, green onions, cilantro, salt and ground red pepper in large bowl. Pour over cheese and noodles. Cover and refrigerate 4 to 6 hours before baking.

3. Preheat oven to 350°F. Bake 50 to 60 minutes or until knife inserted in center comes out clean.

4. Serve with sour cream, avocado or salsa, if desired.

TIP For a spicier flavor, add ¼ to ½ teaspoon chili powder.

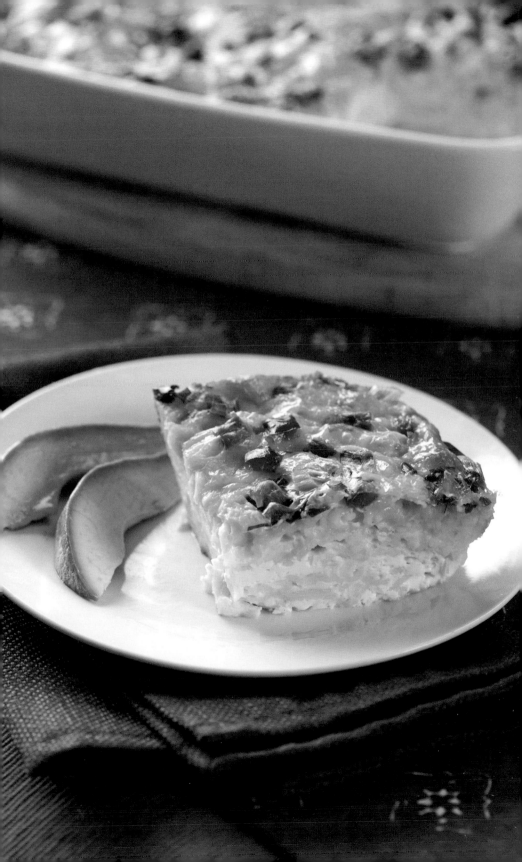

RANCHERO EGGS

MAKES 4 SERVINGS

2 **to 4 fresh serrano chiles***

1 **clove garlic**

1½ **pounds tomatoes, peeled, seeded**

¾ **cup plus 2 tablespoons vegetable oil, divided**

⅓ **cup finely chopped white onion**

¼ **teaspoon salt**

¼ **teaspoon sugar**

¼ **teaspoon ground cumin**

8 **(6-inch) corn tortillas**

8 **eggs**

⅓ **cup dry curd cottage cheese or farmer's cheese**

1 **firm ripe avocado, sliced**

Sprigs fresh cilantro (optional)

Chiles can sting and irritate the skin; wear gloves when handling peppers and do not touch your eyes.

1. Place chiles and garlic in blender; process until finely chopped. Add tomatoes; process until finely chopped, but not smooth.

2. Heat 2 tablespoons oil in medium skillet over medium heat until hot. Add onion. Cook and stir 4 minutes or until onion is softened. Increase heat to medium-high. Stir in tomato mixture, salt, sugar and cumin. Cook and stir 6 to 8 minutes until sauce thickens slightly. Keep warm.

3. Preheat oven to 250°F. Line baking sheet with paper towels. Heat remaining ¾ cup oil in large skillet over medium heat until hot. Fry tortillas, one at a time, in oil 10 to 20 seconds until limp and blistered, turning once. Drain on paper towels. Keep warm in oven on prepared baking sheet.

4. Remove all but 2 tablespoons oil from skillet. Reduce heat to medium-low. Fry eggs, 4 at a time, 2 to 3 minutes until whites are set.

5. Arrange 2 tortillas on each plate; place 1 egg on each tortilla. Top with sauce; sprinkle with cheese. Serve with avocado and cilantro, if desired.

NOTE: For milder flavor, seed some or all of the chiles.

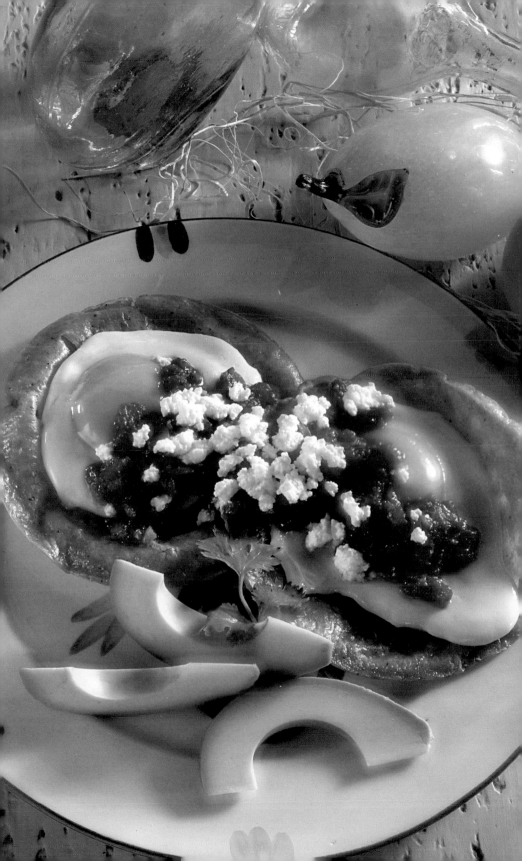

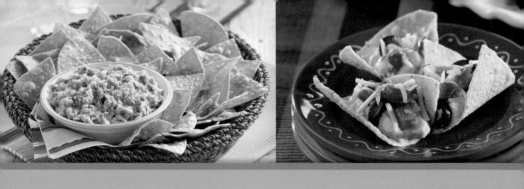

APPETIZERS & SNACKS

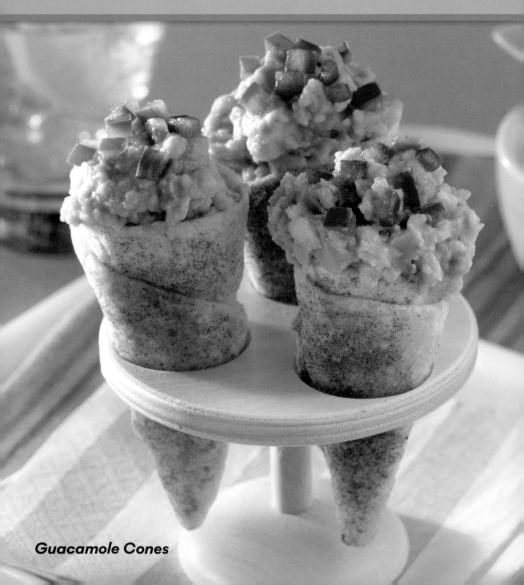

Guacamole Cones

GUACAMOLE CONES

6 (6-inch) flour tortillas
1 tablespoon vegetable oil
1 teaspoon chili powder
2 ripe avocados
1½ tablespoons fresh lime juice
1 tablespoon finely chopped green onion
¼ teaspoon salt
¼ teaspoon black pepper
   Dash hot pepper sauce (optional)
2 to 3 plum tomatoes, chopped

1. Preheat oven to 350°F. Line baking sheet with parchment paper.

2. Cut tortillas in half. Roll each tortilla half into cone shape; secure with toothpick. Brush outside of each cone with oil; sprinkle lightly with chili powder. Place on prepared baking sheet.

3. Bake 9 minutes or until cones are lightly browned. Turn cones upside down; bake about 5 minutes or until golden brown on all sides. Cool cones 1 minute; remove toothpicks and cool completely.

4. Cut avocados in half; remove and discard pits. Scoop avocado pulp from skins and place in medium bowl; mash with fork. Stir in lime juice, green onion, salt, black pepper and hot pepper sauce, if desired, until blended.

5. Place 1 tablespoon chopped tomato in each tortilla cone; top with small scoop of guacamole and additional chopped tomatoes. Serve immediately.

CLASSIC GUACAMOLE

MAKES ABOUT 2 CUPS

4 tablespoons finely chopped white onion, divided

1 to 2 serrano or jalapeño peppers,* seeded and finely chopped

1 tablespoon plus 1½ teaspoons coarsely chopped fresh cilantro, divided

¼ teaspoon chopped garlic (optional)

2 large ripe avocados

1 medium tomato, peeled and chopped

1 to 2 teaspoons fresh lime juice

¼ teaspoon salt

Corn Tortilla Chips (recipe follows) or packaged corn tortilla chips

Serrano and jalapeño peppers can sting and irritate the skin, so wear rubber gloves when handling peppers and do not touch your eyes.

1. Combine 2 tablespoons onion, serrano pepper, 1 tablespoon cilantro and garlic, if desired, in large mortar. Grind with pestle until almost smooth. (Mixture can be processed in food processor, if necessary, but it may become more watery than desired.)

2. Cut avocados lengthwise into halves; remove and discard pits. Scoop out avocado pulp; place in large bowl. Add serrano mixture. Mash roughly, leaving avocado slightly chunky.

3. Add tomato, lime juice, salt, remaining 2 tablespoons onion and 1½ teaspoons cilantro to avocado mixture; mix well. Serve immediately with Corn Tortilla Chips or cover and refrigerate up to 4 hours.

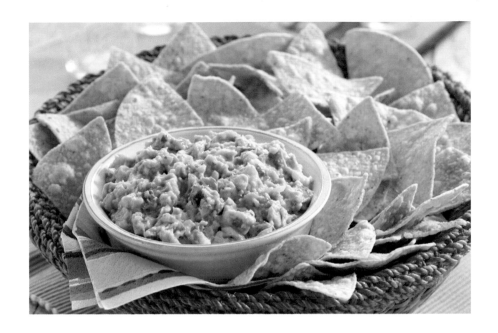

CORN TORTILLA CHIPS

MAKES 6 DOZEN

12 (6-inch) corn tortillas, day-old*

Vegetable oil

½ to 1 teaspoon salt

*If tortillas are fresh, let stand, uncovered, in single layer on wire rack 1 to 2 hours to dry slightly.

1. Stack 6 tortillas. Cutting through stack, cut into 6 equal wedges. Repeat with remaining tortillas.

2. Heat ½ inch oil in large heavy skillet over medium-high heat to 375°F; adjust heat to maintain temperature.

3. Fry tortilla wedges in single layer 1 minute or until crisp, turning occasionally. Remove and drain on paper towels. Sprinkle chips with salt. Repeat with remaining wedges.

TIP Tortilla chips are served with salsa, used as the base for nachos and used as scoops for guacamole, refried beans or other dips. They are best eaten fresh, but can be stored, tightly covered, in cool place 2 to 3 days. Reheat in 350°F oven a few minutes before serving.

7-LAYER DIP

1 package (3 ounces) ramen noodles, any flavor, crushed*

2 tablespoons dried taco seasoning mix

3 ripe avocados, diced

1 jalapeño pepper, finely chopped**

2 tablespoons finely chopped fresh cilantro

2 tablespoons lime juice

1 clove garlic, minced

½ teaspoon salt

1 can (about 15 ounces) refried beans

1 container (16 ounces) sour cream

2 cups (8 ounces) shredded Mexican Cheddar-Jack cheese

2 medium tomatoes, diced

3 green onions, thinly sliced Tortilla chips

*Discard seasoning packet.

**Jalapeño peppers can sting and irritate the skin, so wear rubber gloves when handling peppers and do not touch your eyes.

1. Combine noodles and taco seasoning mix in medium bowl; mix well.

2. Mash avocados, jalapeño pepper, cilantro, lime juice, garlic and salt in large bowl.

3. Spread refried beans in bottom of 8-inch glass baking dish. Layer sour cream, noodles, avocado mixture, cheese, tomatoes and green onions evenly over beans. Serve immediately or cover and refrigerate for up to 8 hours. Serve with tortilla chips.

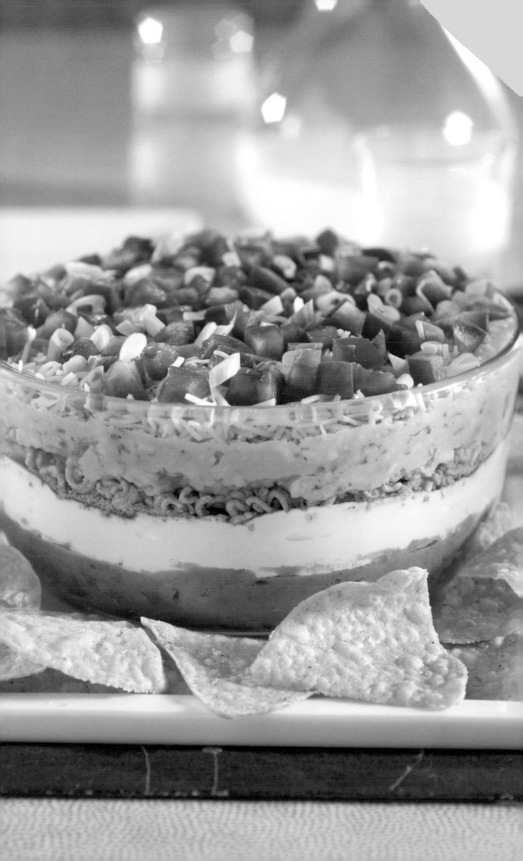

AVOCADO GARDEN MINIS

1 package (3 ounces) oriental-flavored ramen noodles

1 ripe medium avocado, diced

3 tablespoons finely chopped red onion

1 cup grape tomatoes, quartered

¾ cup peeled and diced cucumber

¼ cup chopped fresh cilantro

¼ cup plus 2 tablespoons extra virgin olive oil

2 tablespoons lemon juice

2 medium cloves garlic, minced

¼ teaspoon salt

⅛ teaspoon black pepper

1. Break noodles into 4 pieces. Cook according to package directions using seasoning packet; drain well. Cool.

2. Spoon equal parts of noodles, avocado, onion, tomatoes, cucumber and cilantro into 6 mini mason jars or small ramekins.

3. Whisk oil, lemon juice, garlic, salt and pepper in small bowl. Drizzle dressing over each container. Refrigerate 10 minutes to allow flavors to blend.

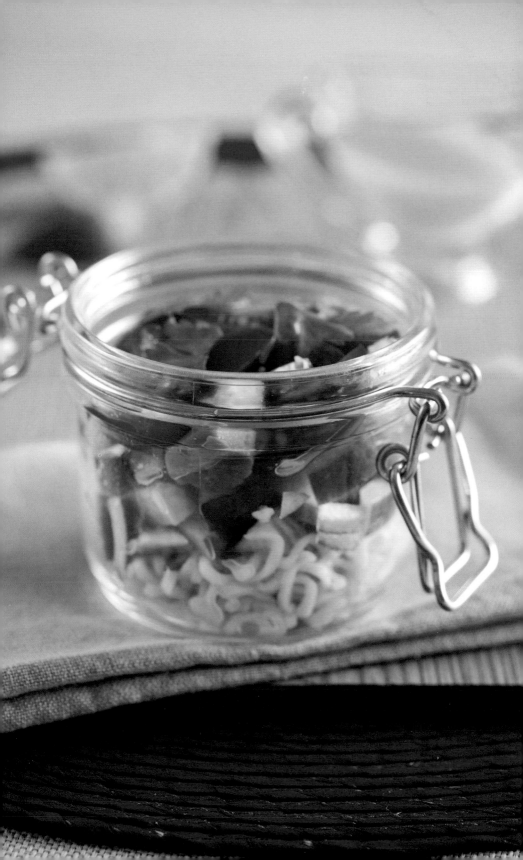

GUACAMOLE SLIDERS

MAKES 12 SMALL BURGERS

1 ripe avocado

1 tablespoon ORTEGA® Fire-Roasted Diced Green Chiles

1 tablespoon chopped cilantro

1 tablespoon lime juice

⅛ teaspoon salt

1 pound lean ground beef

1 tablespoon water

1 cup ORTEGA® Garden Vegetable Salsa, Medium, divided

12 dinner rolls

CUT avocado in half and remove pit. Scoop out avocado with spoon and place in small bowl. Add chiles, cilantro, lime juice and salt. Gently mash with fork until blended; set aside.

COMBINE beef, water and ½ cup salsa in medium bowl. Form mixture into 12 small round balls. Flatten slightly.

GRILL or pan-fry burgers about 3 minutes. Turn over and flatten with spatula. Cook 4 minutes longer or until desired doneness.

CUT each roll in half. Fill with 1 tablespoon remaining salsa, 1 burger and 1 heaping tablespoon guacamole. Serve immediately.

PREP TIME: 10 minutes
START TO FINISH: 20 minutes

TIP Try using a panini press or similar double-sided grill to cook the sliders even faster.

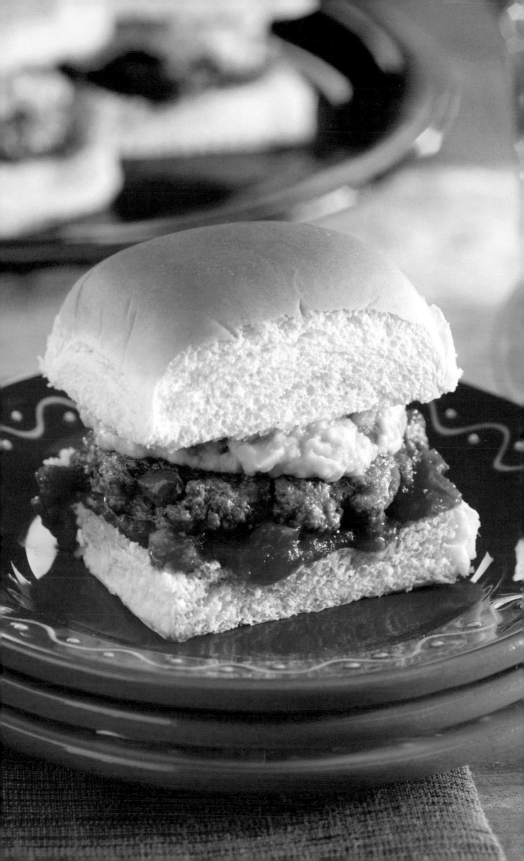

VEGGIE SUSHI ROLLS

MAKES 24 PIECES (ABOUT 4 SERVINGS)

- **2 tablespoons unseasoned rice vinegar**
- **1 teaspoon sugar**
- **½ teaspoon salt**
- **2 cups cooked short grain brown rice**
- **4 sheets sushi nori**
- **1 teaspoon toasted sesame seeds**
- **½ English cucumber, cut into ¼-inch thin pieces**
- **½ red bell pepper, cut into ¼-inch thin pieces**
- **½ ripe avocado, cut into ½-inch thin pieces**
- **Pickled ginger and/or wasabi paste (optional)**

1. Combine vinegar, sugar and salt in large bowl. Stir in rice. Cover with damp towel until ready to use.

2. Prepare small bowl with water and splash of vinegar to rinse fingers and prevent rice from sticking while working. Place 1 sheet of nori horizontally on bamboo sushi mat or waxed or parchment paper, rough side up. Using wet fingers, spread about ½ cup rice evenly over nori, leaving 1-inch border along bottom edge. Sprinkle rice with ¼ teaspoon sesame seeds. Place one fourth of each cucumber, bell pepper and avocado on top of rice.

3. Pick up edge of mat nearest you. Roll mat forward, wrapping rice around fillings and pressing gently to form log; press gently to seal. Place roll on cutting board, seam side down. Repeat with remaining nori and fillings.

4. Slice each roll into 6 pieces using sharp knife.* Cut off ends, if desired. Serve with pickled ginger and/or wasabi, if desired.

*Wipe knife with damp cloth between cuts, if necessary.

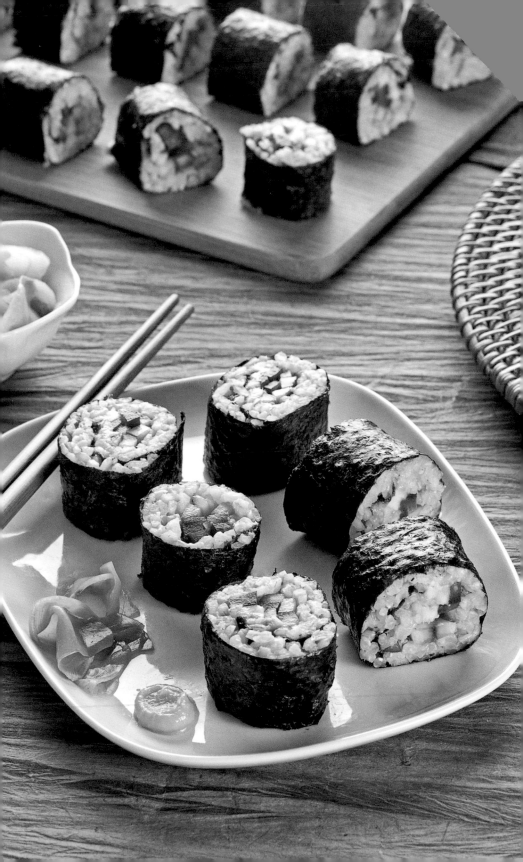

X-MEX GUACAMOLE PLATTER

MAKES 6 TO 8 SERVINGS

4 ripe avocados

¼ cup lime juice

3 cloves garlic, crushed

2 tablespoons olive oil

½ teaspoon salt

¼ teaspoon black pepper

1 cup (4 ounces) shredded Colby Jack cheese

1 cup diced and seeded plum tomatoes

⅓ cup sliced pitted black olives

⅓ cup salsa

1 tablespoon minced fresh cilantro

Tortilla chips

1. Cut avocados in half; remove pits. Scoop out pulp into food processor. Add lime juice, garlic, oil, salt and pepper. Cover; process until almost smooth.

2. Spread avocado mixture evenly onto large dinner plate or serving platter, leaving border around edge. Top with cheese, tomatoes, olives, salsa and cilantro. Serve with tortilla chips.

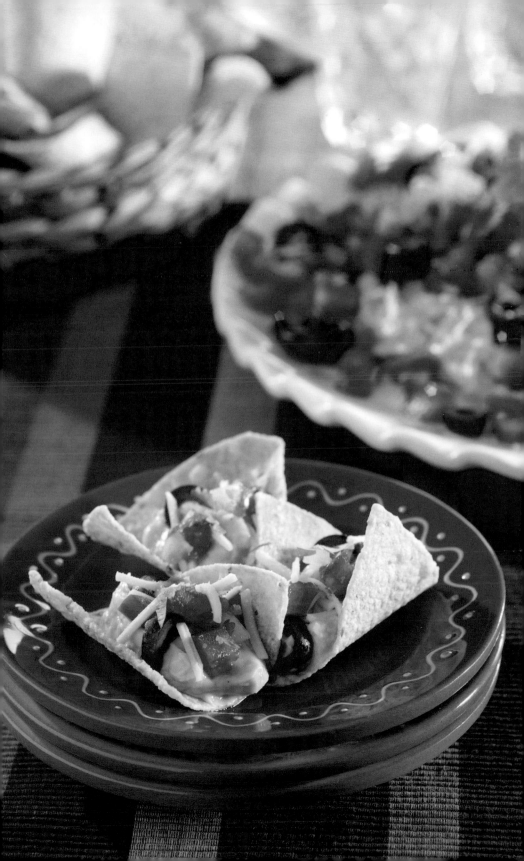

DECONSTRUCTED GAZPACHO IN FIESTA FLATS

1 tomato, diced (about 1 cup)

1 yellow bell pepper, diced (about 1 cup)

1 cup diced cucumber

½ cup green onions, diced

1 cup ORTEGA® Salsa, any variety, divided

1 tablespoon ORTEGA® Taco Seasoning Mix

2 ripe avocados

1 packet (1 ounce) ORTEGA® Guacamole Seasoning Mix

8 ORTEGA® Fiesta Flats Flat Bottom Taco Shells

COMBINE tomatoes, bell pepper, cucumber, green onions, ¼ cup salsa and taco seasoning mix in medium bowl. Mix well to coat vegetables.

CUT each avocado in half; remove pit. Scoop out avocado meat and place in small bowl. Mix with guacamole seasoning mix.

PLACE 1 tablespoon salsa in bottom of each Fiesta Flat. Top each with 2 heaping tablespoons vegetable mixture and dollop of guacamole.

PREP: 15 minutes
START TO FINISH: 15 minutes

TIP The vegetable mixture can rest in the refrigerator overnight to allow the flavors to combine.

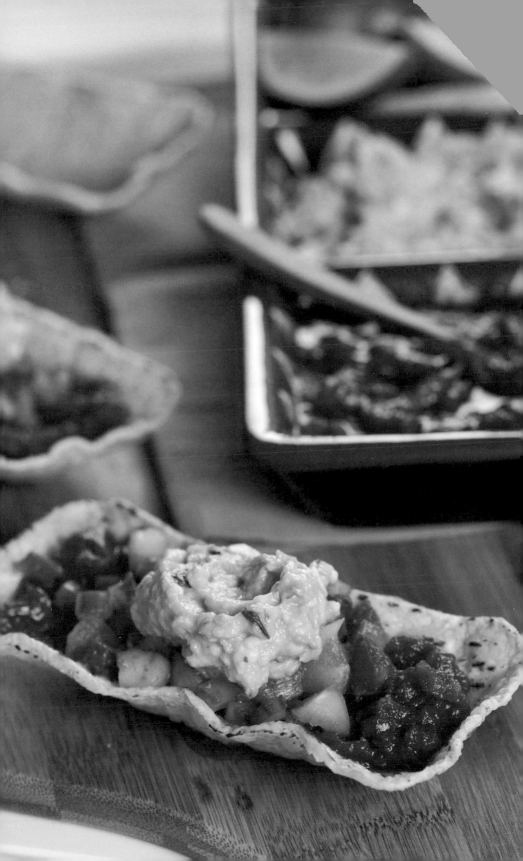

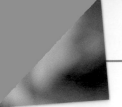

AVOCADO SMASH

MAKES ¾ CUP

1   ripe medium avocado
1   tablespoon lime juice
¼   cup plain nonfat Greek
    yogurt

1   teaspoon Dijon mustard
¼   teaspoon salt
    Chopped fresh chives
    (optional)

Roughly mash avocado with fork in shallow bowl. Stir in remaining ingredients and sprinkle with chives. Serve immediately.

TIP   This dip is great with raw veggies, such as cucumber slices, celery sticks, or red bell pepper strips.

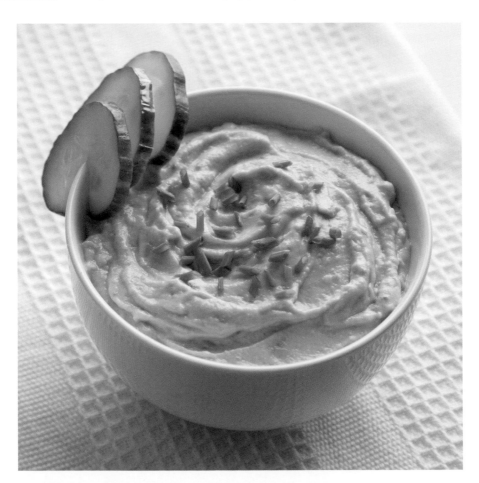

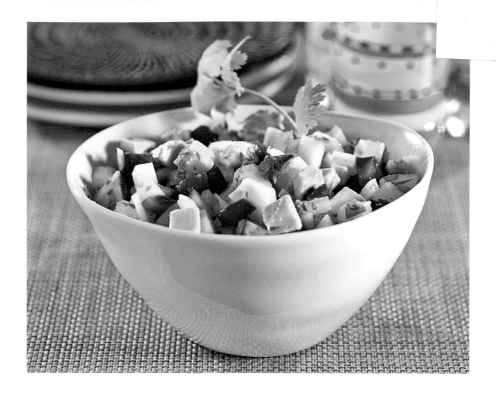

AVOCADO SALSA

MAKES 32 SERVINGS (ABOUT 4 CUPS)

1 medium avocado, diced

1 cup chopped onion

1 cup peeled seeded
chopped cucumber

1 Anaheim pepper,* seeded
and chopped

½ cup chopped fresh tomato

2 tablespoons chopped fresh
cilantro, plus additional
for garnish

½ teaspoon salt

¼ teaspoon hot pepper sauce

*Anaheim peppers can sting and
irritate the skin, so wear rubber
gloves when handling peppers and
do not touch your eyes.*

Combine avocado, onion, cucumber, Anaheim pepper, tomato,
2 tablespoons cilantro, salt and hot pepper sauce in medium bowl;
gently mix. Cover and refrigerate at least 1 hour before serving.
Garnish with additional cilantro.

MEXICAN SHRIMP COCKTAIL

½ cup WISH-BONE® Italian Dressing

1 tomato, chopped

1 can (4 ounces) chopped green chilies, undrained

¼ cup chopped green onions

1½ teaspoons honey

¼ teaspoon hot pepper sauce

1 pound cleaned cooked medium shrimp

1 avocado, peeled and diced

1 tablespoon finely chopped fresh cilantro or parsley

Combine WISH-BONE® Italian Dressing, tomato, chilies, green onions, honey and hot pepper sauce in medium bowl. Stir in shrimp, avocado and cilantro.

TIP Can be made ahead. Stir in avocado, right before serving.

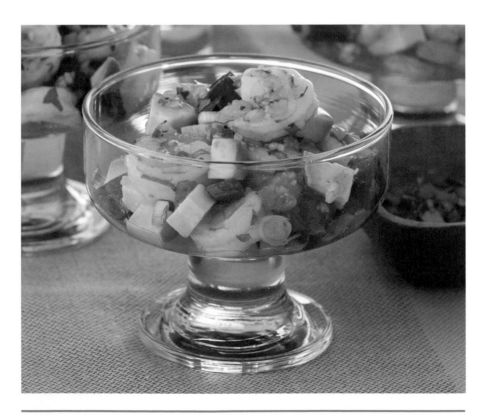

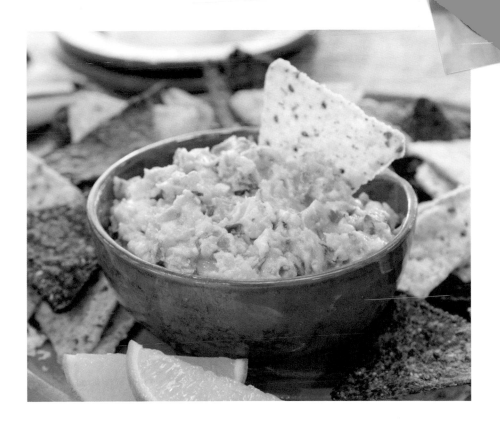

VEGETABLE GUACAMOLE

MAKES 3 CUPS DIP

3 medium avocados, mashed

1 package KNORR® Vegetable recipe mix

¼ cup coarsely chopped canned jalapeño peppers

3 tablespoons chopped fresh cilantro

1 tablespoon lime juice

Combine all ingredients in small bowl; chill if desired. Garnish, if desired, with chopped green onion and serve with tortilla chips or your favorite dippers.

PREP TIME: 10 minutes

SERVING SUGGESTION: A colorful twist on the traditional, this guacamole works well as a dip or an accompaniment to tacos and burritos.

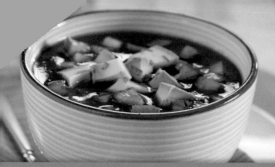
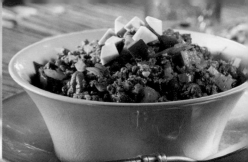

SOUPS, STEWS & CHILIES

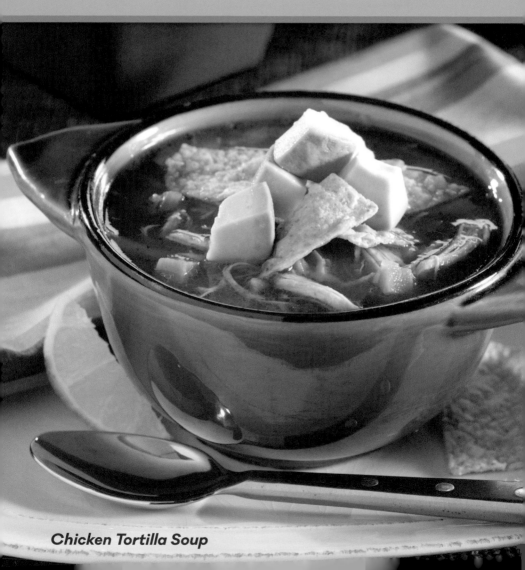

Chicken Tortilla Soup

CHICKEN TORTILLA SOUP

2 tablespoons canola oil

½ cup finely chopped onion

½ cup finely chopped carrot

2½ cups shredded cooked rotisserie chicken

1 cup thick and chunky salsa

4 cups chicken broth

1 tablespoon lime juice

1 avocado, chopped

10 corn tortilla chips, broken into thirds

1. Heat oil in large saucepan over high heat. Add onion and carrot; cook and stir 3 minutes or until onion is translucent.

2. Stir in chicken and salsa. Add broth; bring to a boil. Reduce heat to medium-low; cover and simmer 5 minutes or until carrot is crisp-tender. Remove from heat; stir in lime juice.

3. Top with avocado and tortilla chips before serving.

RED & GREEN NO-BEAN CHILI

4 pounds ground beef

2 large onions, chopped

3 banana peppers, seeded and sliced

¼ cup chili powder

2 tablespoons minced garlic

1 can (about 28 ounces) diced tomatoes with mild green chiles, undrained

1 can (about 14 ounces) beef broth

2 cans (4 ounces each) diced mild green chiles, drained

2 tablespoons ground cumin

2 tablespoons cider or malt vinegar

1 to 2 tablespoons hot paprika

1 tablespoon dried oregano

Hot pepper sauce

Diced avocado and red onions

1. Brown beef in large skillet or Dutch oven over medium-high heat 6 to 8 minutes, stirring to break up meat. Drain fat. Stir in onions, banana peppers, chili powder and garlic. Reduce heat to medium-low; cook 30 minutes, stirring occasionally.

2. Add tomatoes, broth, green chiles, cumin, vinegar, paprika, oregano and hot pepper sauce. Cook 30 minutes, stirring occasionally. Garnish with avocado and red onions.

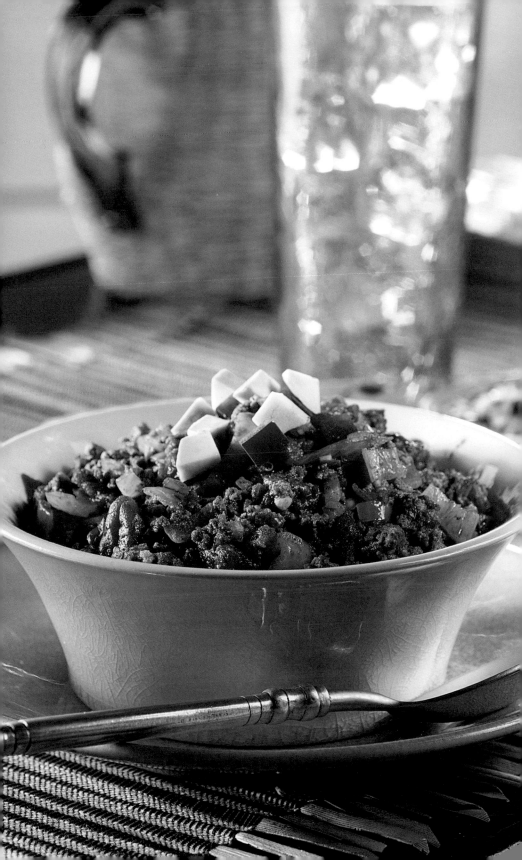

CHILE VERDE CHICKEN STEW

⅓ cup all-purpose flour

1½ teaspoons salt, divided

¼ teaspoon black pepper

1½ pounds boneless skinless chicken breasts, cut into 1½-inch pieces

4 tablespoons vegetable oil, divided

1 pound tomatillos (about 9), husked and halved

2 onions, chopped

2 cans (4 ounces each) diced mild green chiles

1 tablespoon dried oregano

1 tablespoon ground cumin

2 cloves garlic, chopped

1 teaspoon sugar

2 cups reduced-sodium chicken broth

8 ounces Mexican beer

5 red potatoes, diced

Chopped fresh cilantro, sour cream, shredded Monterey Jack cheese, lime wedges, diced avocado and/or hot pepper sauce (optional)

1. Combine flour, 1 teaspoon salt and pepper in large bowl. Add chicken; toss to coat. Heat 2 tablespoons oil in large nonstick skillet over medium heat. Add chicken; cook until lightly browned on all sides, stirring occasionally. Transfer to Dutch oven.

2. Heat remaining 2 tablespoons oil in same skillet. Stir in tomatillos, onions, chiles, oregano, cumin, garlic, sugar and remaining ½ teaspoon salt. Cook and stir 20 minutes or until vegetables are softened. Stir in broth and beer. Working in batches, process mixture in food processor or blender until almost smooth.

3. Add mixture to chicken in Dutch oven. Stir in potatoes. Cover; bring to a boil over medium-high heat. Reduce heat to low; simmer 1 hour or until potatoes are tender, stirring occasionally. Garnish each serving with cilantro and other toppings, as desired.

VARIATION: Omit potato and serve over hot white rice.

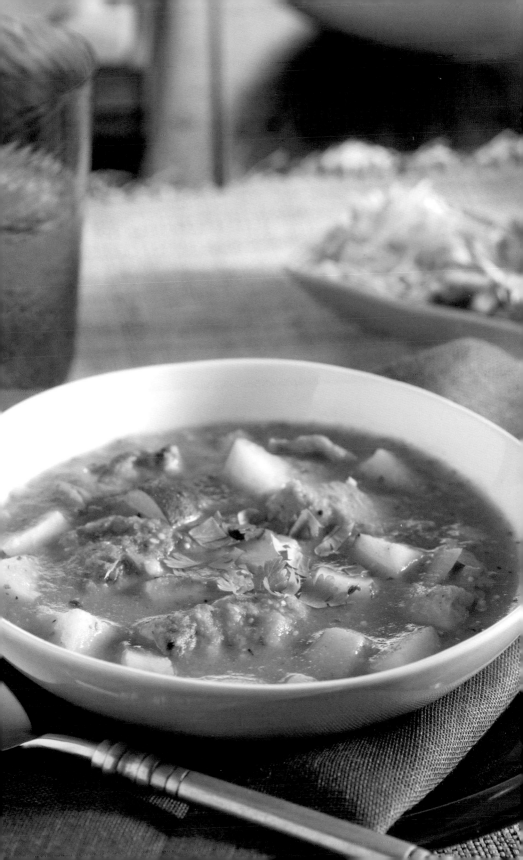

GAZPACHO

6 large very ripe tomatoes (about 3 pounds), divided

1½ cups tomato juice

1 clove garlic

2 tablespoons fresh lime juice

2 tablespoons olive oil

1 tablespoon white wine vinegar

1 teaspoon sugar

½ to 1 teaspoon salt

½ teaspoon dried oregano

6 green onions, sliced

¼ cup finely chopped celery

¼ cup finely chopped seeded cucumber

1 or 2 fresh jalapeño peppers,* seeded, minced

Garlic Croutons (recipe follows) or packaged croutons (optional)

1 cup diced avocado

1 red or green bell pepper, chopped

2 tablespoons chopped fresh cilantro

Lime wedges and sour cream (optional)

Jalapeño peppers can sting and irritate the skin, so wear rubber gloves when handling peppers and do not touch your eyes.

1. Seed and finely chop 1 tomato; set aside.

2. Coarsely chop remaining 5 tomatoes; process half of tomatoes, ¾ cup tomato juice and garlic in blender until smooth. Press through sieve into large bowl; discard seeds. Repeat with remaining coarsely chopped tomatoes and ¾ cup tomato juice.

3. Whisk lime juice, oil, vinegar, sugar, salt and oregano into tomato mixture. Stir in finely chopped tomato, onions, celery, cucumber and jalapeño pepper. Cover; refrigerate at least 4 hours or up to 24 hours to develop flavors.

4. Prepare Garlic Croutons, if desired. Stir soup; ladle into chilled bowls. Top with croutons, avocado, bell pepper and cilantro. Serve with lime wedges and sour cream.

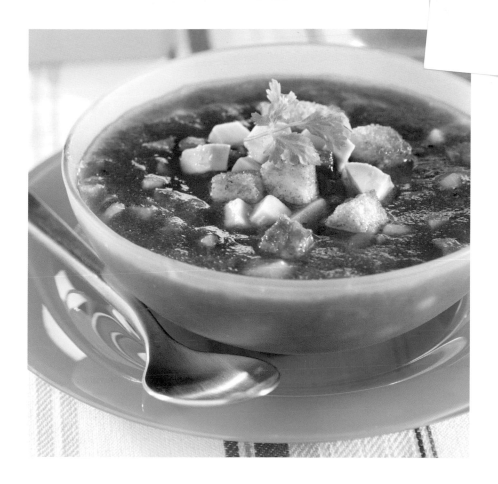

GARLIC CROUTONS

MAKES ABOUT 2 CUPS

5 slices firm white bread	1 clove garlic, minced
2 tablespoons olive oil	¼ teaspoon paprika

1. Preheat oven to 300°F. Trim crusts from bread; cut into ½-inch cubes.

2. Heat oil in skillet over medium heat. Stir in garlic and paprika. Add bread; cook and stir 1 minute just until bread is evenly coated with oil.

3. Spread bread on baking sheet. Bake 20 to 25 minutes until crisp and golden. Cool.

MEXICAN ROASTED GARLIC SOUP

MAKES 4 SERVINGS

3   large whole garlic heads

2   tablespoons olive oil

¾   teaspoon salt

1   tablespoon butter

1   tablespoon all-purpose
    flour

1   can (14.5 ounces) chicken
    broth

2   cups water

1   can (4 ounces) ORTEGA®
    Fire-Roasted Diced Green
    Chiles

¼   teaspoon ground red
    pepper

4   green onions, diced

1   avocado, diced

1   ORTEGA® Flour Soft
    Tortilla, cut into thin
    strips

PREHEAT oven to 400°F.

CUT tops off garlic heads to expose tops of cloves. Drizzle evenly with olive oil and sprinkle with salt. Wrap each head in aluminum foil; place on cookie sheet. Bake 1 hour or until very tender. Remove from pan; cool 10 minutes or until cool enough to handle. Unwrap; squeeze garlic from bottom of heads into small saucepan. Discard skins.

ADD butter and flour. Whisk over medium heat 3 minutes or until garlic sizzles and flour browns slightly. Add half of broth; bring to a boil. Whisk until thickened; add 2 cups water and remaining broth. Reduce heat; simmer 5 minutes. Stir in chiles and red pepper; cook 5 minutes longer.

SERVE in bowls with green onions and avocado. Garnish with tortilla strips.

PREP TIME: 15 minutes

START TO FINISH: 1 hour 20 minutes

TIP   For an authentic, hearty Mexican chicken soup, stir in shredded cooked chicken while simmering.

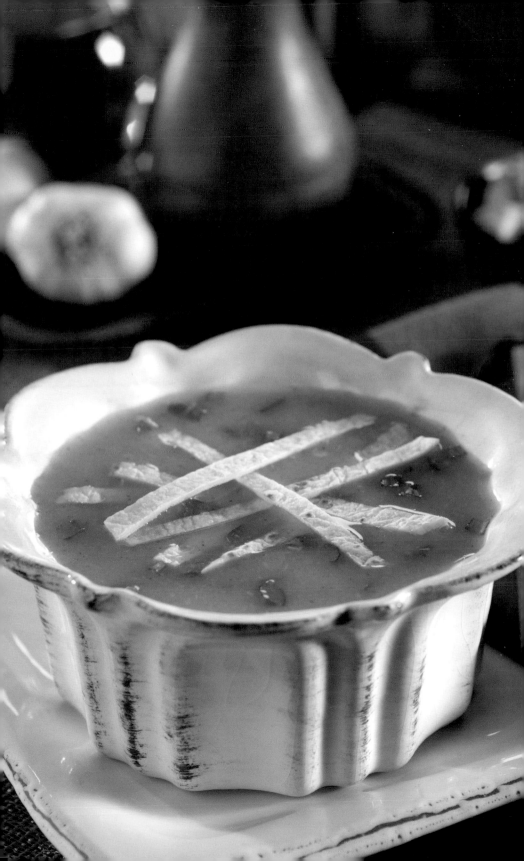

CHILLED AVOCADO SOUP

1 **small onion, sliced ¼ inch thick, divided**

1 **can (about 14 ounces) chicken broth**

½ **cup plain yogurt**

1½ **tablespoons lemon juice**

1 **large ripe avocado, halved**

3 **to 5 drops hot pepper sauce**

Salt

White pepper

¼ **cup finely chopped tomato**

¼ **cup finely chopped cucumber**

Sprigs fresh cilantro

1. Place 1 onion slice, broth, yogurt and lemon juice in blender or food processor container fitted with metal blade; process until well blended. Remove pulp from avocado; spoon into blender. Process until smooth. Pour into bowl. Add hot pepper sauce, salt and pepper. Finely chop remaining onion slices; add to soup. Stir in tomato and cucumber.

2. Cover and refrigerate 2 hours or up to 24 hours. Serve cold. Garnish with cilantro and additional chopped tomato and cucumber, if desired.

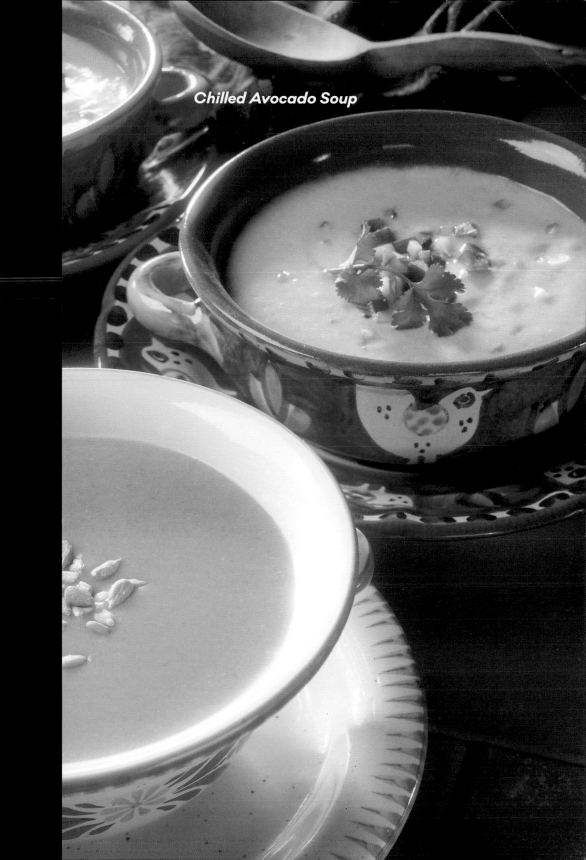
Chilled Avocado Soup

TORTILLA SOUP

MAKES 4 SERVINGS

Vegetable oil

3 (6- or 7-inch) corn tortillas, halved and cut into strips

½ cup chopped onion

1 clove garlic, minced

2 cans (about 14 ounces each) chicken broth

1 can (about 14 ounces) diced tomatoes

1 cup shredded cooked chicken

2 teaspoons fresh lime juice

1 small avocado, diced

2 tablespoons fresh cilantro

1. Pour oil to depth of ½ inch in small skillet. Heat over medium-high heat until oil reaches 360°F on deep-fry thermometer. Add tortilla strips, a few at a time, fry 1 minute or until crisp and lightly browned. Remove with slotted spoon; drain on paper towels.

2. Heat 2 teaspoons oil in large saucepan over medium heat. Add onion and garlic; cook and stir until onion is soft. Add broth and tomatoes; bring to a boil. Cover; reduce heat and simmer 15 minutes.

3. Add chicken and lime juice; simmer 5 minutes. Top soup with tortilla strips, avocado and cilantro.

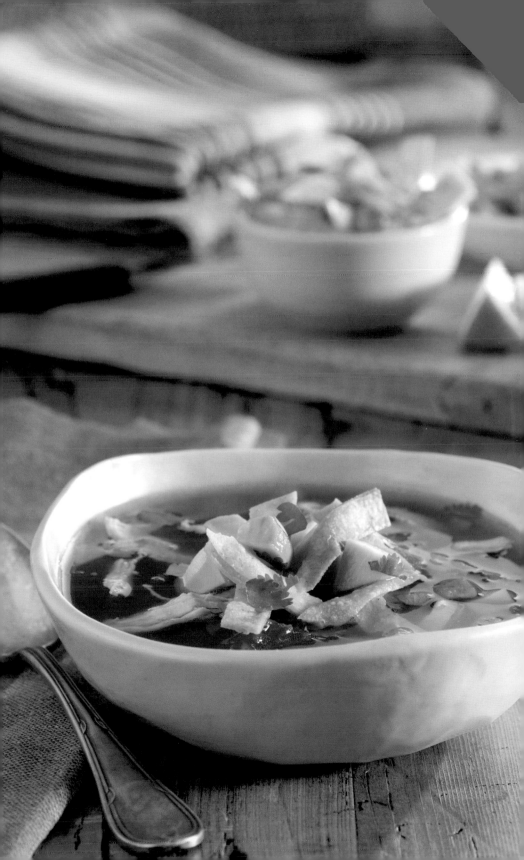

UMMER'S BEST GAZPACHO

3 cups tomato juice

2½ cups finely diced tomatoes (2 large)

1 cup finely diced yellow or red bell pepper (1 small)

1 cup finely diced unpeeled cucumber

½ cup chunky salsa

1 tablespoon olive oil

1 clove garlic, minced

1 ripe avocado, diced

¼ cup finely chopped fresh cilantro or basil

1. Combine tomato juice, tomatoes, bell pepper, cucumber, salsa, oil and garlic in large bowl; mix well. Cover and chill at least 1 hour or up to 24 hours before serving.

2. Stir in avocado and cilantro just before serving.

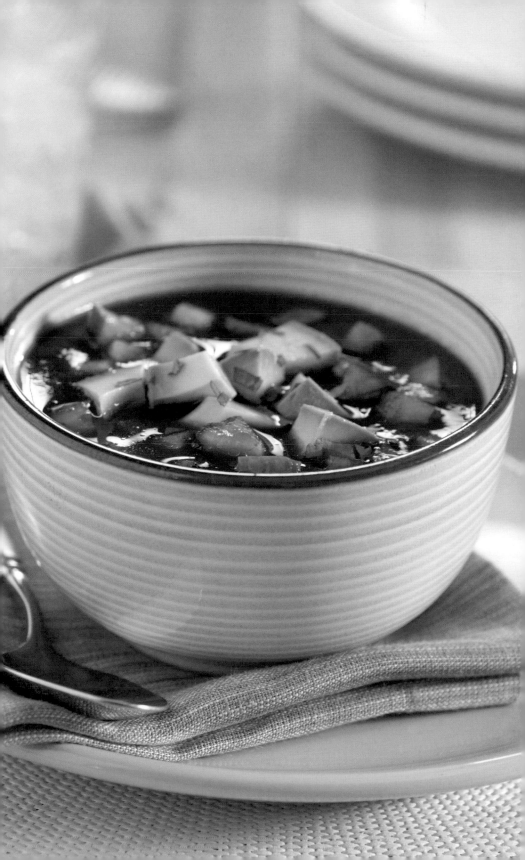

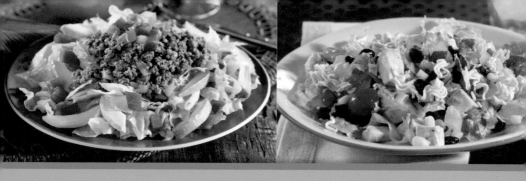

SALADS & SIDES

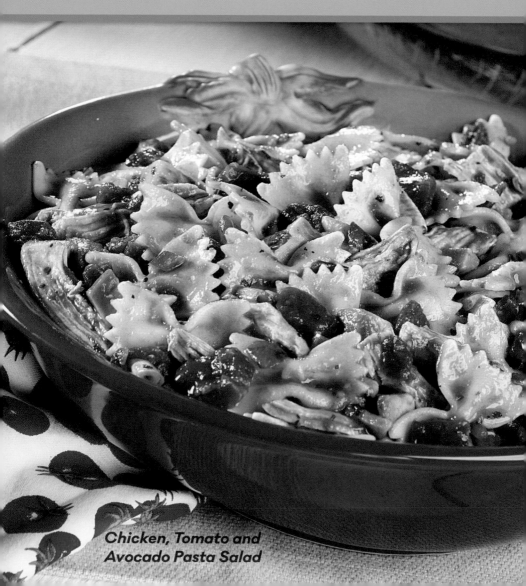

Chicken, Tomato and Avocado Pasta Salad

CHICKEN, TOMATO AND AVOCADO PASTA SALAD

2 cans (14.5 ounces each) HUNT'S® Diced Tomatoes with Balsamic Vinegar, Basil & Olive Oil, undrained

4 cups shredded cooked chicken *Soy meat*

2 medium avocados, pitted, diced

4 green onions, sliced

1 box (16 ounces) farfalle pasta, cooked according to package directions, drained, kept warm

¼ cup finely chopped walnuts (optional)

COMBINE tomatoes, chicken, avocados and onions in a medium saucepan; simmer 10 minutes.

TOSS tomato mixture with warm pasta in a large serving dish.

SPRINKLE with walnuts, if desired.

PREP TIME: 15 minutes
COOK TIME: 20 minutes

SHRIMP AND NO-COOK COUSCOUS SALAD

MAKES 6 SERVINGS

2 cups water

1 box (10 ounces) dry couscous

1 pound frozen cooked shrimp, thawed and patted dry

1 medium cucumber, peeled, seeded and diced

1 medium poblano chile pepper,* seeded and chopped

2 ripe medium avocados, coarsely chopped (about 3/4-inch pieces)

1/2 cup chopped red bell pepper

1 can (2 1/4 ounces) sliced black olives, drained

1/4 cup chopped fresh cilantro or to taste

1/4 cup extra virgin olive oil

1 teaspoon grated lime peel

6 tablespoons lime juice (from 3 medium limes)

2 teaspoons salt

1/8 teaspoon red pepper flakes

3 large tomatoes, sliced (optional)

*Chili peppers can sting and irritate the skin, so wear rubber gloves when handling peppers and do not touch your eyes.

1. Heat water to boiling. Place couscous in large bowl. Pour boiling water over couscous. Cover bowl with plastic wrap. Let stand 5 minutes or until water is absorbed. Fluff with fork. Cool to room temperature. (To cool quickly, spread couscous in a thin layer on a baking sheet or platter.)

2. Place remaining ingredients, except tomatoes, with cooked couscous in same large bowl. Toss well. Serve immediately or refrigerate 2 hours before serving. Serve on bed of lettuce or sliced tomatoes, if desired.

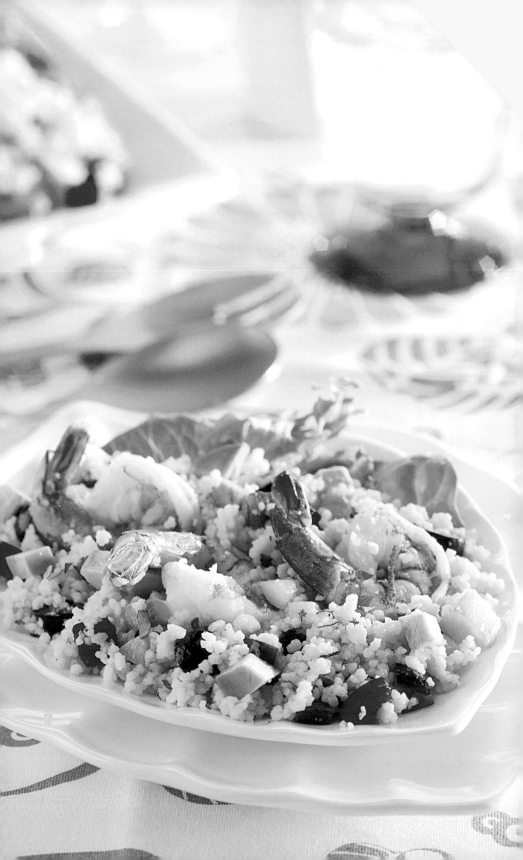

LAYERED MEXICAN SALAD

1 package (10 ounces) shredded lettuce

½ cup chopped green onions (green and white parts)

½ cup sour cream

⅓ cup medium picante sauce

1 medium lime, halved

1 teaspoon sugar

½ teaspoon ground cumin

1 medium avocado, chopped

¾ cup (3 ounces) shredded sharp Cheddar cheese

2 ounces baked tortilla chips, coarsely crumbled

1. Place lettuce evenly in 13×9-inch baking dish. Sprinkle with green onions.

2. Stir together sour cream, picante sauce, juice from half of lime, sugar and cumin in small bowl. Spoon evenly over lettuce and green onions. Place avocado evenly over sour cream layer. Squeeze remaining lime half evenly over avocado layer. Sprinkle evenly with cheese.

3. Cover with plastic wrap. Refrigerate until serving. (May be prepared 8 hours in advance, if desired.) Sprinkle with crumbled tortilla chips before serving.

VARIATION: Add chopped fresh tomatoes to avocado layer. Sprinkle chip layer with chopped fresh cilantro.

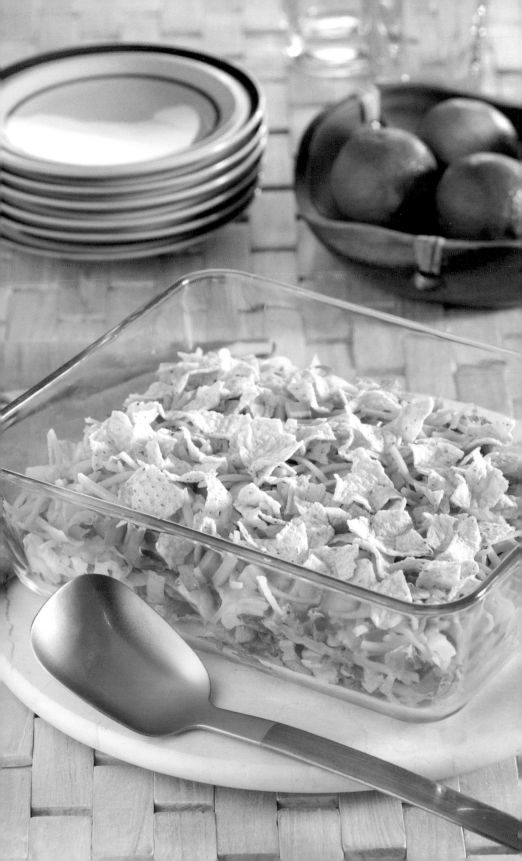

TACO SALAD

MAKES 4 SERVINGS

1 pound ground beef
1 small onion, finely chopped
1 clove garlic, minced
2 teaspoons chili powder
1 teaspoon ground cumin
½ teaspoon salt
   Dash black pepper

1 large head iceberg lettuce, torn into bite-size pieces (about 10 cups)
2 large tomatoes, chopped
1 medium avocado, sliced
2 cups salsa

1. Brown ground beef in medium skillet; drain. Add onion and garlic; cook until tender. Stir in seasonings.

2. Combine lettuce, tomatoes and avocado in large serving bowl; toss lightly. Top with ground beef mixture. Serve with salsa.

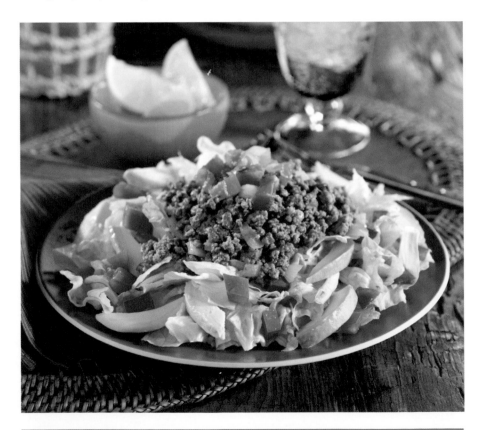

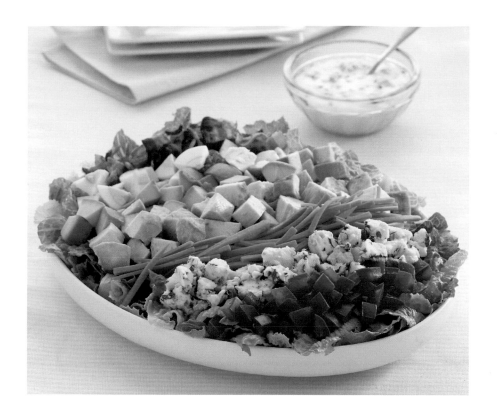

COBB SALAD

MAKES 4 SERVINGS

1 package (10 ounces) torn mixed salad greens *or* 8 cups torn romaine lettuce

6 ounces cooked chicken breast, cut into bite-size pieces

1 tomato, seeded and chopped

2 hard-cooked eggs, cut into bite-size pieces

4 slices bacon, crisp-cooked and crumbled

1 ripe avocado, diced

1 large carrot, shredded

½ cup blue cheese, crumbled

Blue cheese dressing (optional)

1. Place lettuce in serving bowl. Arrange chicken, tomato, eggs, bacon, avocado, carrot and cheese on top of lettuce.

2. Serve with dressing, if desired.

SANTA FE BBQ RANCH SALAD

MAKES 4 SERVINGS

1 cup CATTLEMEN'S® Golden Honey Barbecue Sauce, divided

½ cup ranch salad dressing

1 pound boneless, skinless chicken

12 cups washed and torn Romaine lettuce

1 small red onion, thinly sliced

1 small ripe avocado, diced ½-inch

4 ripe plum tomatoes, sliced

2 cups shredded Monterey Jack cheese

½ cup cooked, crumbled bacon

1. Prepare BBQ Ranch Dressing: Combine ½ cup barbecue sauce and salad dressing in small bowl; reserve.

2. Grill or broil chicken over medium-high heat 10 minutes until no longer pink in center. Cut into strips and toss with remaining ½ cup barbecue sauce.

3. Toss lettuce, onion, avocado, tomatoes, cheese and bacon in large bowl. Portion on salad plates, dividing evenly. Top with chicken and serve with BBQ Ranch Dressing.

PREP TIME: 15 minutes
COOK TIME: 10 minutes

TIP Serve *CATTLEMEN'S*® Golden Honey Barbecue Sauce as a dipping sauce with chicken nuggets or seafood kabobs.

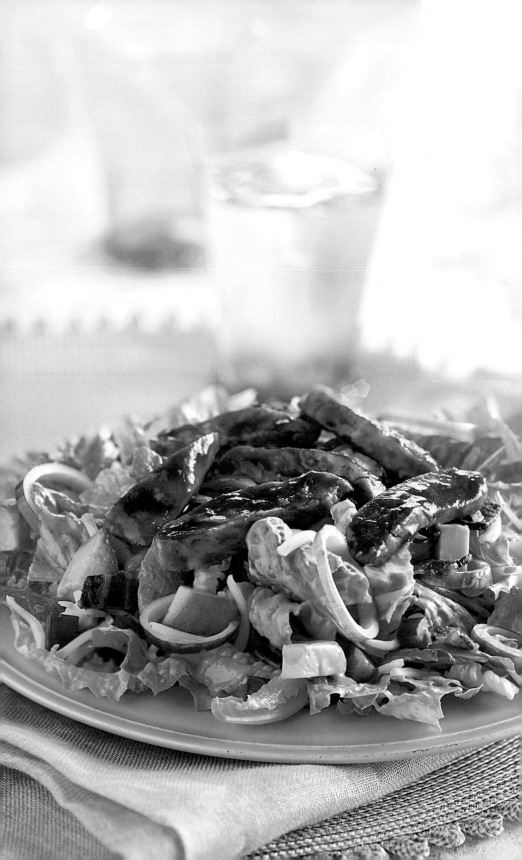

CALIFORNIA CHICKEN AND PASTA SALAD

1⅓ cups uncooked penne pasta

8 ounces chicken breast, cooked and diced (about 2 cups) *Soy Chick*

1 large stalk celery, thinly sliced

1 green onion, trimmed and chopped

1 tablespoon minced cilantro

DRESSING

⅓ cup orange juice

¼ teaspoon curry powder

¼ teaspoon salt

⅛ teaspoon black pepper

1 tablespoon white wine vinegar

1 teaspoon canola oil

¼ cup diced avocado

1. Cook pasta according to package directions, omitting salt; drain. Combine pasta, chicken, celery, green onion and cilantro in large serving bowl.

2. In small bowl, combine orange juice, curry powder, salt, pepper, vinegar and oil. Stir well.

3. Pour dressing over salad and toss well. Add avocado and toss gently.

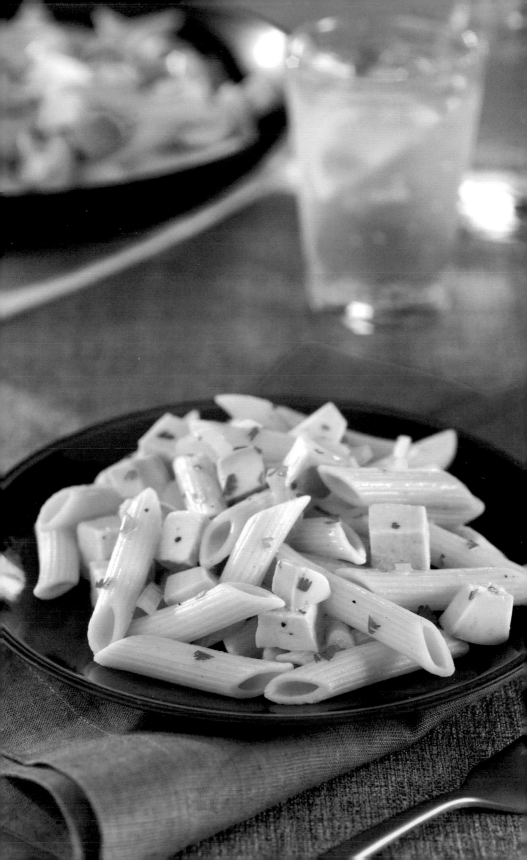

ACAPULCO AVOCADO SALAD

MAKES 4 SERVINGS

Lettuce leaves

2 tablespoons REGINA® White Wine Vinegar

2 tablespoons olive oil

1 mango, diced

½ pound medium shrimp (26- to 30-count), cooked, peeled, deveined, cut in half

1 can (4 ounces) ORTEGA® Diced Green Chiles, drained

½ cup ORTEGA® Salsa, any variety

2 ripe avocados

ARRANGE lettuce on four plates. Set aside.

COMBINE vinegar and oil in medium bowl; mix well. Stir in mango, shrimp, chiles and salsa.

CUT avocados in half and remove pits. Using spoon, scoop some avocado flesh from pit area of each half. Chop and gently stir into shrimp mixture.

REMOVE remainder of avocado from skin; run spoon between flesh and skin, and carefully scoop out avocado halves in one piece. Place each half on lettuce bed.

SPOON shrimp mixture evenly into avocado halves.

PREP TIME: 10 minutes
START TO FINISH: 20 minutes

TIP
To prepare an avocado, insert a sharp knife into the stem end. Slice in half lengthwise to the pit, turning the avocado while slicing. Remove the knife blade and twist the halves in opposite directions to pull apart. Press the knife blade into the pit, twisting the knife gently to pull the pit away from the avocado. Discard pit.

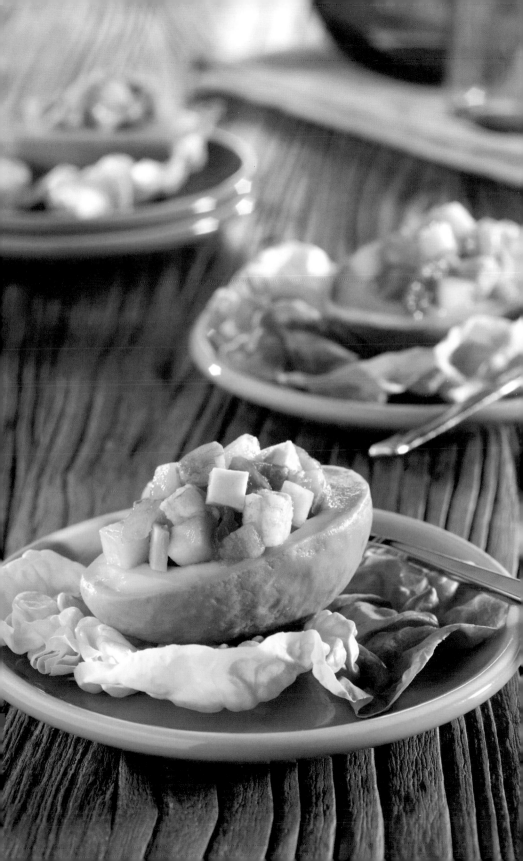

GAZPACHO SHRIMP SALAD

MAKES 4 SERVINGS

½ cup chunky salsa

1 tablespoon balsamic vinegar

1 tablespoon extra virgin olive oil

1 clove garlic, minced

8 cups torn mixed salad greens or romaine lettuce

1 large tomato, chopped

1 small ripe avocado, diced

½ cup thinly sliced unpeeled cucumber

½ pound large cooked shrimp, peeled and deveined

½ cup coarsely chopped fresh cilantro

1. Combine salsa, vinegar, oil and garlic in small bowl; blend well.

2. Combine greens, tomato, avocado and cucumber in large bowl. Evenly divide salad among 4 plates; top with shrimp. Drizzle dressing over salads. Sprinkle with cilantro.

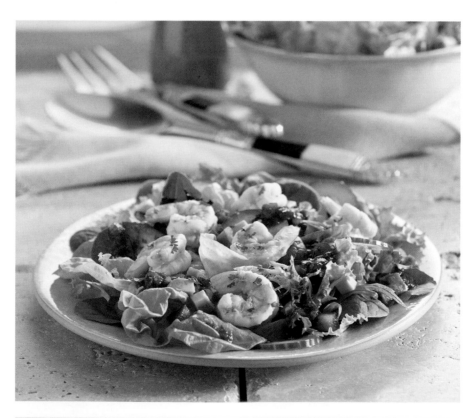

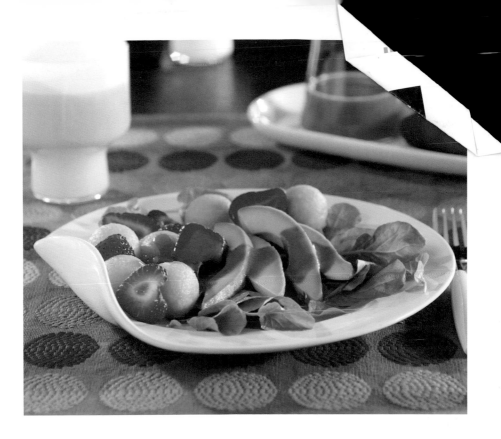

FABULOUS FRUIT SALAD WITH STRAWBERRY VINAIGRETTE

MAKES 4 SERVINGS

2 cups fresh strawberry
  slices, divided

3 tablespoons vegetable oil

2 tablespoons lime juice

2 tablespoons red wine
  vinegar

1 teaspoon sugar

1 bunch watercress, trimmed

2 avocados, sliced

2 cups cantaloupe balls

1. Combine 1 cup strawberry slices, oil, lime juice, vinegar and sugar in food processor; process until smooth. Strain mixture through fine-mesh sieve; discard solids.

2. Arrange watercress on plates; top with avocados, cantaloupe and remaining 1 cup strawberries. Drizzle with vinaigrette.

...STY ZUCCHINI-CHICKPEA SALAD

MAKES 4 TO 6 SERVINGS

3 medium zucchini (about 6 ounces each)

½ teaspoon salt

5 tablespoons white vinegar

1 clove garlic, minced

¼ teaspoon dried thyme

½ cup olive oil

1 cup drained canned chickpeas

½ cup sliced pitted black olives

3 green onions, minced

1 canned chipotle pepper in adobo sauce, drained, seeded, minced

1 ripe avocado, cut into ½-inch cubes

⅓ cup crumbled feta *or* 3 tablespoons grated Romano cheese

1 head Boston lettuce, cored, separated into leaves

Sliced tomatoes and sprigs fresh cilantro (optional)

1. Cut zucchini lengthwise into halves; cut halves crosswise into ¼-inch-thick slices. Place slices in medium bowl; sprinkle with salt. Toss to mix. Spread zucchini on several layers of paper towels. Let stand at room temperature 30 minutes to drain.

2. Combine vinegar, garlic and thyme in large bowl. Gradually add oil, whisking continuously until dressing is thoroughly blended.

3. Pat zucchini dry; add to dressing. Add chickpeas, olives and green onions; toss lightly to coat. Cover and refrigerate at least 30 minutes or up to 4 hours, stirring occasionally.

4. Add chipotle pepper to salad just before serving. Stir gently to mix. Add avocado and cheese; toss lightly to mix.

5. Serve salad in lettuce-lined shallow bowl or plate. Garnish, if desired.

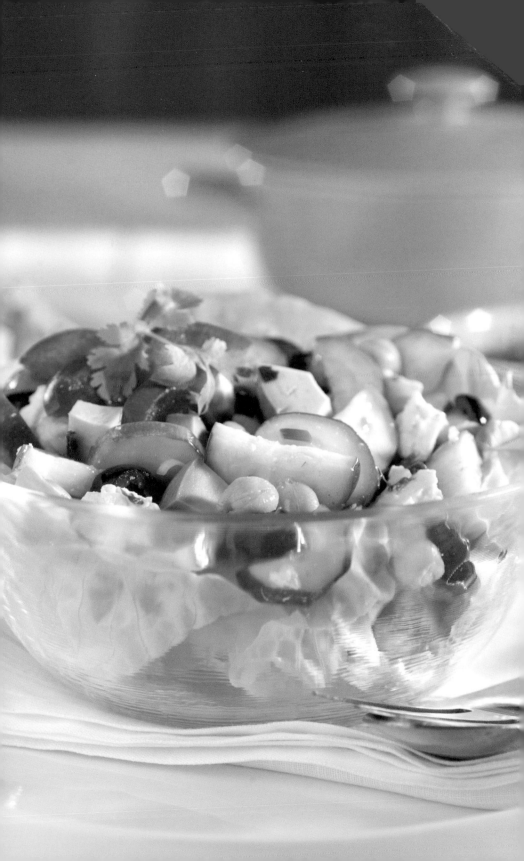

CRAB SALAD TOSTADAS

- 2 (6-inch) tortillas
- 2 tablespoons mayonnaise
- 1 tablespoon fresh lime juice
- 2 teaspoons minced fresh jalapeño pepper*
- 2 cups packed mixed field or baby greens
- ½ cup diced tomato
- 2 tablespoons minced cilantro
- 2 tablespoons finely diced red onion
- 1 can (6 ounces) all white ~~crabmeat, drained~~ *Tuna?*
- ½ cup diced ripe avocado

*Jalapeño peppers can sting and irritate the skin, so wear rubber gloves when handling peppers and do not touch your eyes.

1. Heat oven to 400°F. Place tortillas on baking sheet coated with nonstick cooking spray. Bake 6 minutes or until crisp and golden brown.

2. Meanwhile, mix mayonnaise, lime juice and jalapeño pepper in large bowl. Add greens, tomato, cilantro and onion; toss well. Add crabmeat and avocado; toss again. Serve on tortillas.

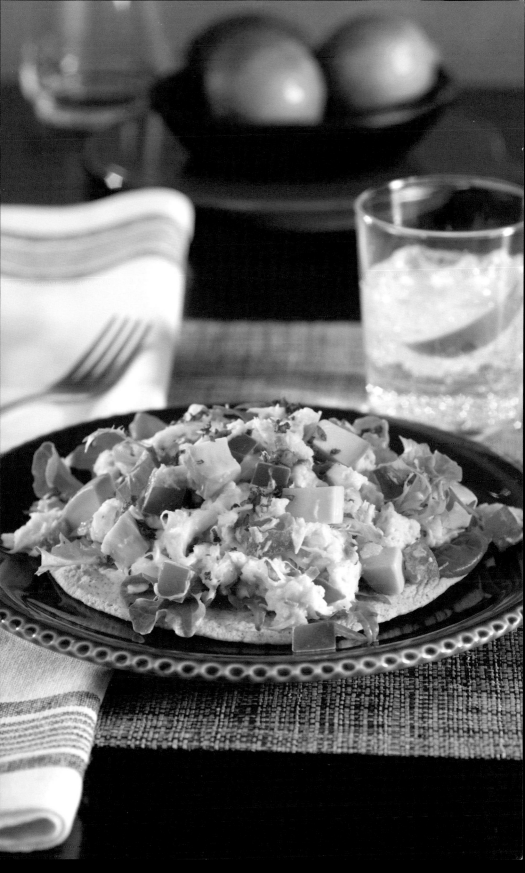

SOUTHWESTERN SALAD

2 hearts of romaine lettuce, cut crosswise into ½-inch-thick strips

1 cup frozen corn, thawed

1 cup halved cherry tomatoes

8 ounces boneless skinless chicken breasts, cooked and diced

1 ripe avocado, diced

1 red bell pepper, diced

1 can (about 15 ounces) black beans, rinsed and drained

DRESSING

1½ tablespoons minced shallot

¼ cup lime juice

2 teaspoons honey

⅓ cup olive oil

½ teaspoon kosher salt

¼ teaspoon black pepper

2 tablespoons finely chopped fresh cilantro (optional)

1 package (3 ounces) ramen noodles, any flavor, broken into small pieces*

Discard seasoning packet.

1. Combine romaine, corn, tomatoes, chicken, avocado, bell pepper and beans in large bowl; toss well.

2. Whisk shallot, lime juice, honey, oil, salt, black pepper and cilantro, if desired, in medium bowl. Add to salad mixture; toss to coat. Sprinkle with noodles.

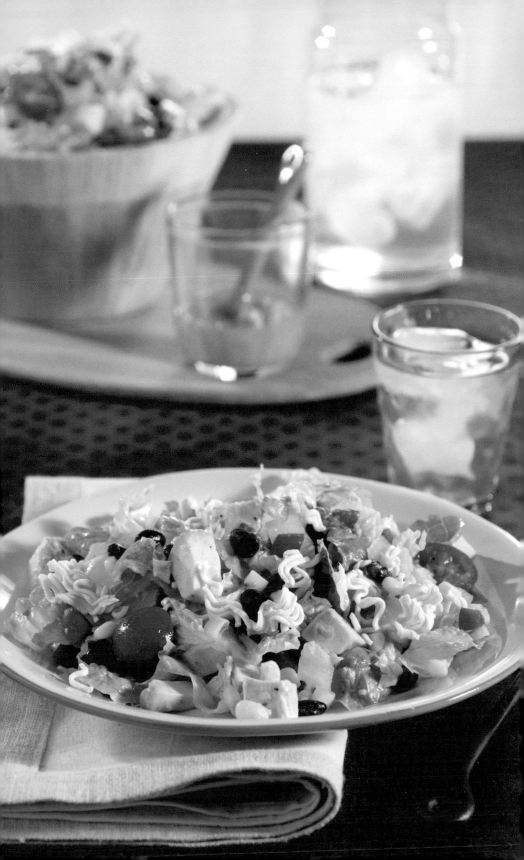

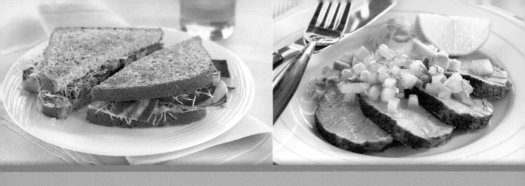

DINNERS & SANDWICHES

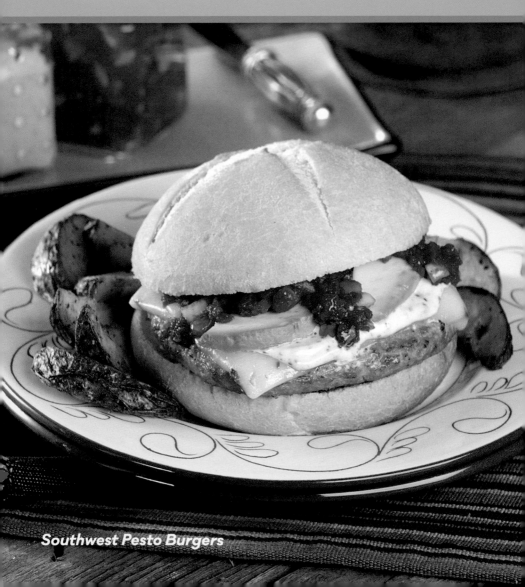

Southwest Pesto Burgers

SOUTHWEST PESTO BURGERS

½ cup fresh cilantro, stemmed

1½ teaspoons chopped jalapeño pepper*

1 clove garlic

¾ teaspoon salt, divided

¼ cup vegetable oil

2 tablespoons light or regular mayonnaise

1¼ pounds ground beef

4 slices pepper jack cheese

4 Kaiser rolls, split

1 ripe avocado, sliced

Salsa

*Jalapeño peppers can sting and irritate the skin, so wear rubber gloves when handling peppers and do not touch your eyes.

1. Combine cilantro, jalapeño pepper, garlic and ¼ teaspoon salt in food processor; process until garlic is minced. With motor running, slowly add oil through feed tube; process until thick paste forms. Combine mayonnaise and 1 tablespoon pesto in small bowl; mix well.

2. Prepare grill for direct cooking. Combine beef, remaining ¼ cup pesto and ½ teaspoon salt in large bowl; mix lightly. Shape into 4 patties.

3. Grill over medium heat, covered, 8 to 10 minutes (or uncovered, 13 to 15 minutes) or until cooked through (160°F), turning occasionally. Top with cheese during last minute of grilling.

4. Place patties on bottom halves of rolls; top with mayonnaise mixture, avocado, salsa and top halves of rolls.

PORK TENDERLOIN WITH AVOCADO-TOMATILLO SALSA

MAKES 4 SERVINGS

1½ teaspoons chili powder

½ teaspoon ground cumin

1 pound pork tenderloin

1 teaspoon extra virgin olive oil

SALSA

2 medium tomatillos, husked and diced*

½ ripe medium avocado, diced

1 jalapeño pepper,** seeded and finely chopped

1 clove garlic, minced

2 tablespoons finely chopped red onion

1 tablespoon lime juice

1 to 2 tablespoons chopped fresh cilantro

⅛ teaspoon salt

4 lime wedges (optional)

*Remove the husk by pulling from the bottom to where it attaches at the stem. Wash before using.

**Jalapeño peppers can sting and irritate the skin, so wear rubber gloves when handling and do not touch your eyes.

1. Preheat oven to 425°F. Combine chili powder and cumin in small bowl. Sprinkle evenly on pork, pressing to allow spices to adhere.

2. Heat oil in large nonstick skillet over medium-high heat until hot. Add pork and cook 3 minutes. Turn; cook 2 to 3 minutes longer or until richly browned. Place on foil-lined baking sheet; bake 20 to 25 minutes or until barely pink in center (about 165°F). Remove from oven and let stand 5 minutes before slicing.

3. Combine salsa ingredients in small bowl and toss gently to blend. Serve with pork slices and additional lime wedges, if desired.

TIP Choose firm tomatillos with dry husks that are not too ragged. Store in a paper bag in refrigerator for up to a month.

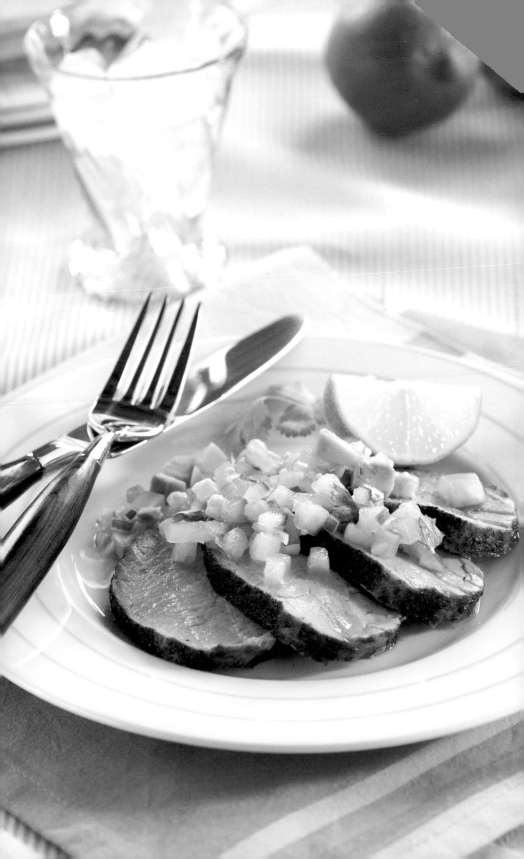

2 tablespoons FRENCH'S®
   Honey Dijon Mustard

2 tablespoons mayonnaise

2 tablespoons sour cream

~~1 pound ground beef~~

2 tablespoons FRENCH'S®
   Worcestershire Sauce

1⅓ cups FRENCH'S® Cheddar
    or Original French Fried
    Onions, divided

½ teaspoon garlic salt

¼ teaspoon ground black
   pepper

4 hamburger rolls, split and
   toasted

½ small avocado, sliced

½ cup sprouts

Beyond Beef
or
Beast meat patty

1. Combine mustard, mayonnaise and sour cream; set aside.

2. Combine beef, Worcestershire, ⅔ cup French Fried Onions and
   seasonings. Form into 4 patties. Grill over high heat until juices run
   clear (160°F internal temperature).

3. Place burgers on rolls. Top each with mustard sauce, avocado
   slices, sprouts and remaining onions, dividing evenly. Cover with
   top halves of rolls.

PREP TIME: 10 minutes
COOK TIME: 10 minutes

BBQ CHEESE BURGERS: Top each burger with 1 slice American
cheese, 1 tablespoon barbecue sauce and 2 tablespoons French
Fried Onions.

PIZZA BURGERS: Top each burger with pizza sauce, mozzarella
cheese and French Fried Onions.

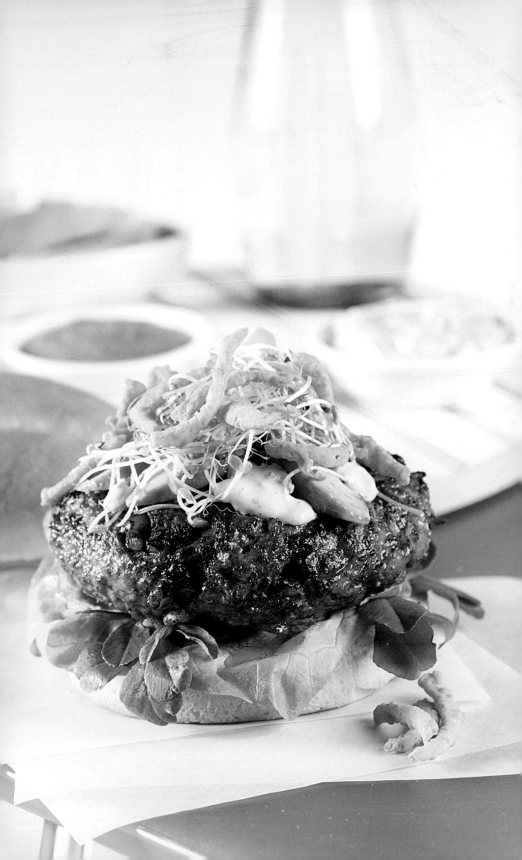

SHRIMP AND AVOCADO TOSTADAS

1 cup canned refried beans

8 ounces medium raw shrimp, peeled and deveined

3 cloves garlic, minced

3 green onions, sliced

½ cup salsa

1 ripe avocado, diced

4 tostada shells, warmed

½ cup shredded romaine lettuce

½ cup diced tomato

1. Heat small saucepan over medium heat; add refried beans and cook until heated through.

2. Meanwhile, spray large nonstick skillet with nonstick cooking spray; heat over medium-high heat. Add shrimp and garlic; cook and stir 3 minutes or until shrimp are pink and opaque. Add green onions; cook and stir 30 seconds. Stir in salsa; cook until heated through. Remove from heat; gently stir in avocado.

3. Spread beans evenly over tostada shells; top with shrimp mixture, lettuce and tomato.

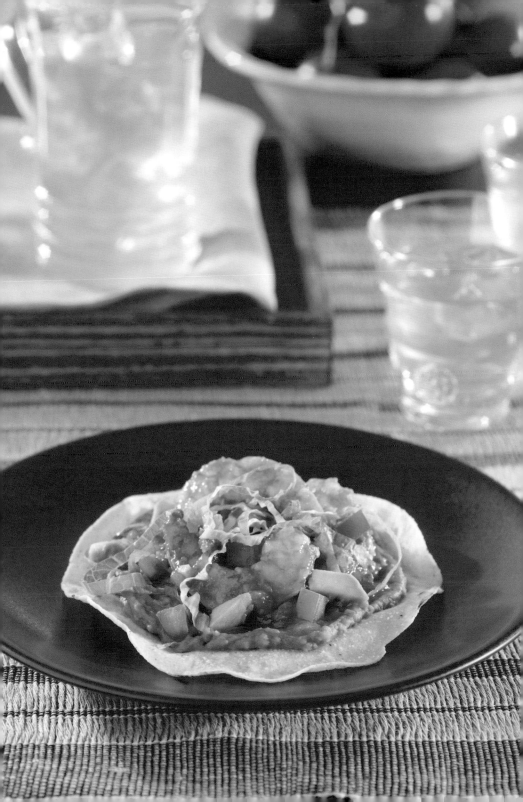

TOASTED COBB SALAD SANDWICHES

MAKES 2 SANDWICHES

½ medium avocado

1 green onion, chopped

½ teaspoon lemon juice
Salt and black pepper

2 Kaiser rolls, split

4 ounces thinly sliced deli chicken or turkey

4 slices bacon crisp-cooked

1 hard-cooked egg, sliced

2 slices (1 ounce each) Cheddar cheese

½ cup blue cheese
Tomato slices (optional)
Olive oil

1. Mash avocado in small bowl; stir in green onion and lemon juice. Season with salt and pepper. Spread avocado mixture on cut sides of roll tops.

2. Layer bottoms of rolls with chicken, bacon, egg, Cheddar cheese, blue cheese and tomato, if desired. Close sandwiches with roll tops. Brush outsides of sandwiches lightly with olive oil.

3. Heat large nonstick skillet over medium heat. Add sandwiches; cook 4 to 5 minutes per side or until cheese melts and sandwiches are golden brown.

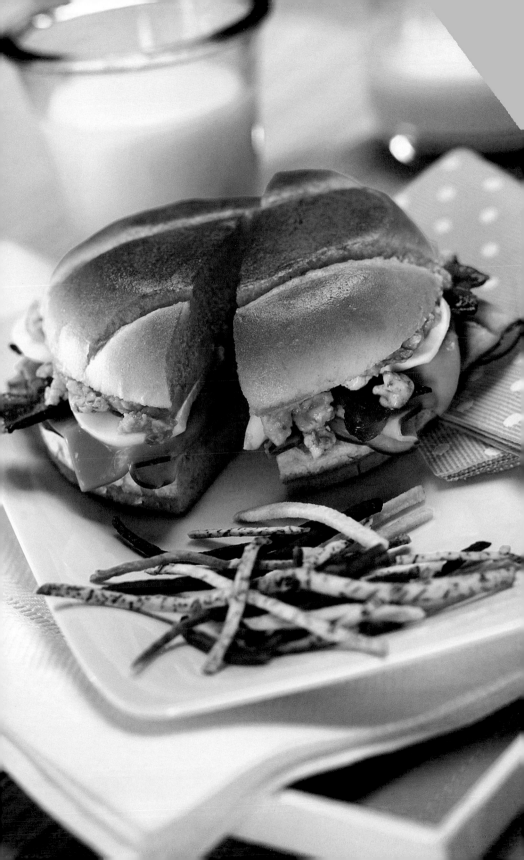

MAKES 4 SERVINGS

drained lenti Soup

2 **cups water**

¾ **cup dried green lentils, rinsed and sorted**

2 **cloves garlic, minced**

1 **teaspoon chili powder**

1 **teaspoon ground cumin**

⅛ **teaspoon ground red pepper**

⅓ **cup plain dry bread crumbs**

¼ **cup finely chopped fresh cilantro or green onions**

3 **egg whites**

2 **teaspoons canola oil**

4 **whole wheat hamburger buns, split and lightly toasted**

⅓ **cup salsa**

½ **ripe avocado, sliced**

1. Combine water and lentils in medium saucepan. Bring to a boil over high heat. Reduce heat; cover and simmer 20 minutes or until lentils are tender. Drain well in a strainer. (Do not rinse.)

2. With motor running, drop garlic cloves through feed tube of food processor; process until minced. Add 1¼ cups lentils, chili powder, cumin and ground red pepper; process until lentils are minced.

3. Place remaining lentils in large bowl. Add bread crumbs, cilantro, egg whites and minced lentil mixture. Mix well; shape into 4 patties about 4 inches in diameter. Cover; refrigerate at least 30 minutes or up to 2 hours.

4. Heat oil in large nonstick skillet over medium heat. Add patties; cook 5 minutes per side or until golden brown. Serve on buns topped with salsa and avocado.

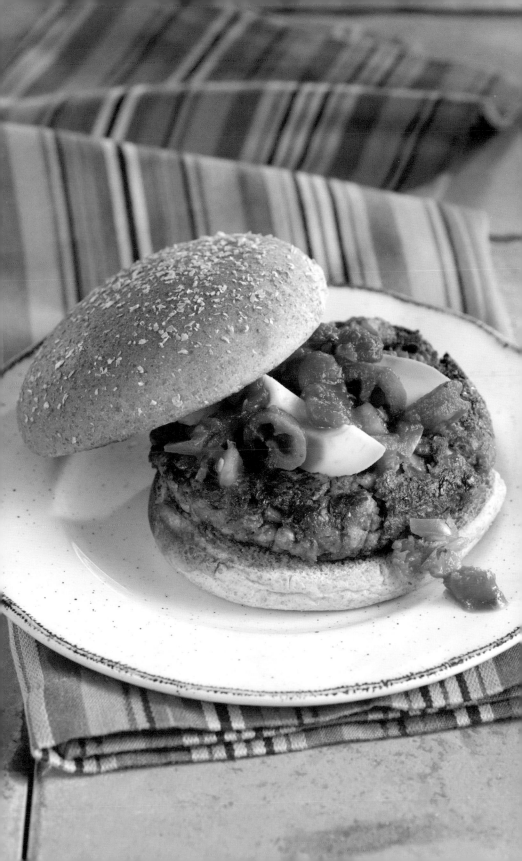

BACON AND AVOCADO SANDWICHES

MAKES 4 SERVINGS

12 slices vegetarian bacon

½ ripe avocado

2 tablespoons plain reduced-fat yogurt

1 teaspoon fresh lemon juice

8 thin slices whole wheat sandwich bread, toasted

8 slices tomato

1 cup alfalfa sprouts

1. Cook bacon according to package directions.

2. Combine avocado, yogurt and lemon juice in small bowl; stir with fork until smooth. Spread about 1 tablespoon avocado mixture on 1 side of 4 bread slices.

3. Top each with 3 slices bacon, 2 slices tomato, ¼ cup alfalfa sprouts and remaining bread slice.

TIP Once peeled, the pulp of an avocado begins to discolor almost immediately. Lightly brush the cut surfaces of the fruit with lemon or lime juice to prevent them from darkening.

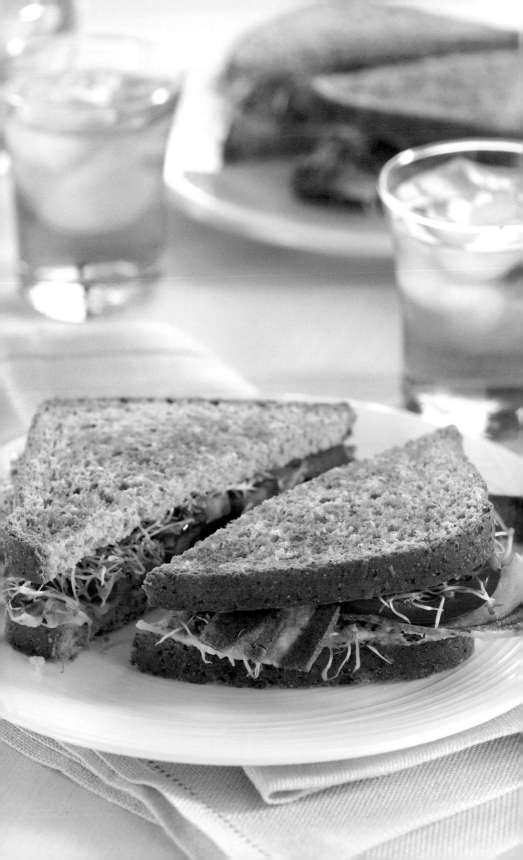

GRILLED CHICKEN WITH CORN AND BLACK BEAN SALSA

MAKES 4 SERVINGS

- ½ cup corn
- ½ cup finely chopped red bell pepper
- ½ of a 15-ounce can black beans, rinsed and drained
- ½ ripe medium avocado, diced
- ¼ cup chopped fresh cilantro
- 2 tablespoons fresh lime juice
- 1 tablespoon chopped sliced pickled jalapeño pepper
- ½ teaspoon salt, divided
- 1 teaspoon black pepper
- ½ teaspoon chili powder
- 4 boneless skinless chicken breasts (4 ounces each), pounded to ½-inch thickness

1. Combine corn, bell pepper, beans, avocado, cilantro, lime juice, jalapeño pepper and ¼ teaspoon salt in medium bowl. Set aside.

2. Combine black pepper, remaining ¼ teaspoon salt and chili powder in small bowl; sprinkle over chicken.

3. Coat grill pan with nonstick cooking spray. Cook chicken over medium-high heat 4 minutes per side or until no longer pink in center.

4. Serve chicken topped with salsa.

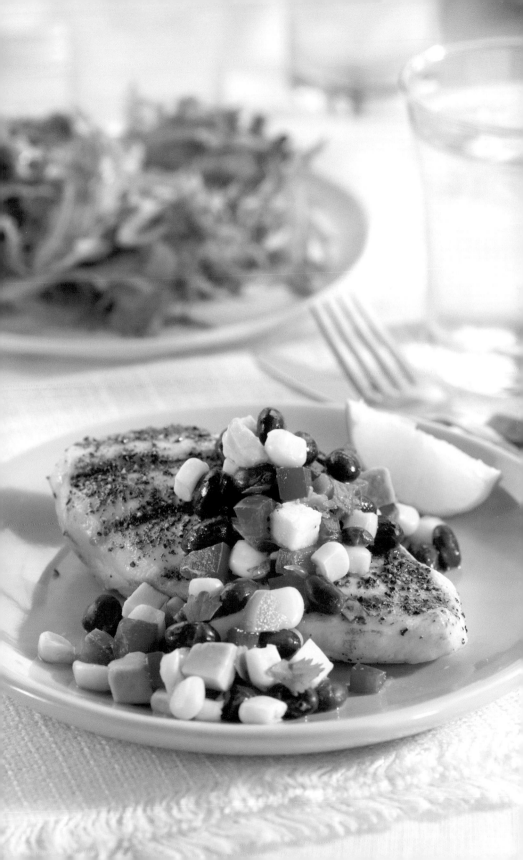

CHIPOTLE SHRIMP TACOS

1 packet (1.25 ounces) ORTEGA® Chipotle Seasoning Mix

32 large shrimp (about 1½ pounds), peeled, deveined

1 teaspoon olive oil

8 ORTEGA® Yellow Corn Taco Shells

2 cups shredded iceberg lettuce

1 ripe avocado, cut into 16 slices

¾ cup ORTEGA® Salsa Verde

PLACE seasoning mix in large bowl. Add shrimp; toss to coat well.

HEAT oil in large nonstick skillet over medium-high heat until hot. Add shrimp. Cook 1½ minutes on each side or just until done. (Do not overcook.) Remove from heat.

HEAT taco shells in microwave according to package directions. Place 2 taco shells on each of 4 plates. Fill each shell with 4 shrimp, ¼ cup lettuce, 2 avocado slices and 1½ tablespoons salsa.

PREP TIME: 5 minutes
START TO FINISH: 15 minutes

TIP You can easily slice an avocado half right in the skin. Use the tip of a knife to make slices inside the peel, then gently scoop them out with a spoon.

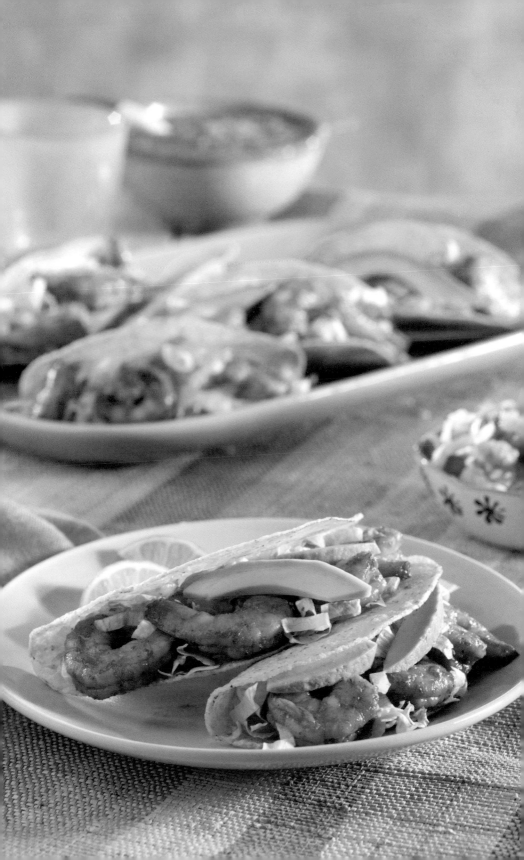

MEXICALI TORTILLA SKILLET

12 ounces lean ground beef

2 medium poblano peppers, seeded and chopped

1 cup diced onion

12 ounces ripe tomatoes, chopped (about 3 medium)

1 tablespoon ground cumin

2 teaspoons paprika

2 to 3 teaspoons sugar

½ teaspoon salt

2 ounces baked tortilla chips, coarsely crumbled

¼ cup (1 ounce) shredded sharp Cheddar cheese

½ ripe medium avocado, chopped

¼ cup chopped fresh cilantro

¼ cup sour cream

1 lime, quartered

1. Cook and stir beef in large nonstick skillet over medium-high heat 2 minutes. Stir in peppers and onion; cook and stir 4 minutes or until soft. Stir in tomatoes, cumin, paprika and sugar; bring to a boil. Reduce heat; cover and simmer 5 to 10 minutes or until tomatoes are tender. Remove from heat; stir in salt.

2. Top with tortilla chips, cheese, avocado and cilantro. Serve with sour cream and lime wedges.

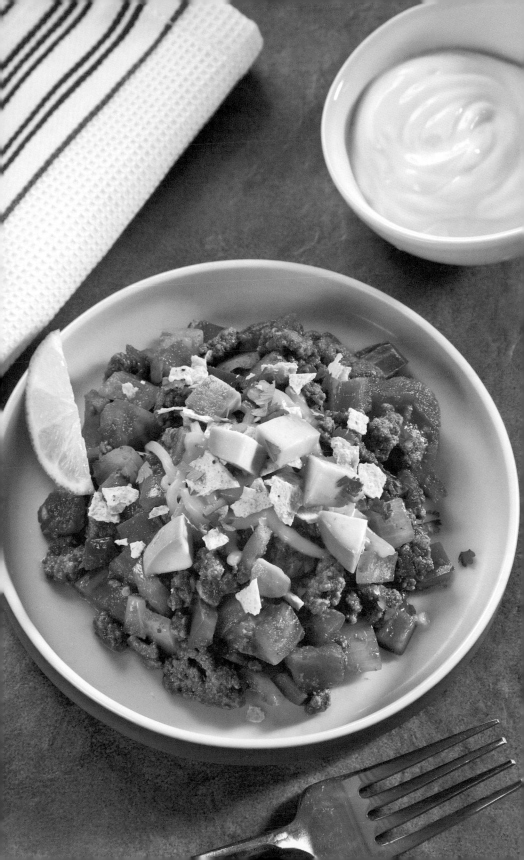

DEVIL'S FIRE SHREDDED BEEF TACOS

MAKES 6 TO 8 SERVINGS

1 boneless beef chuck roast (2½ pounds)

1¼ teaspoons salt, divided

1 teaspoon *each* cumin, garlic powder and smoked paprika

2 tablespoons olive oil, divided

2 cups beef broth

1 red bell pepper, sliced

1 tomato, cut into wedges

½ onion, sliced

2 cloves garlic, minced

1 to 2 canned chipotle peppers in adobo sauce

Juice of 1 lime

Corn or flour tortillas

Optional toppings: sliced bell peppers, avocado, diced onion, lime wedges and/or chopped fresh cilantro

1. Season beef with 1 teaspoon salt, cumin, garlic powder and smoked paprika. Heat 1 tablespoon oil in large skillet over medium-high heat. Add beef; cook 5 minutes on each side until browned. Remove to slow cooker.

2. Pour in broth. Cover; cook on LOW 8 to 9 hours or on HIGH 4 to 5 hours.

3. Meanwhile, preheat oven to 425°F. Combine bell pepper, tomato, onion and garlic on large baking sheet. Drizzle with remaining 1 tablespoon oil. Roast 40 minutes or until vegetables are tender. Place vegetables, chipotle pepper, lime juice and remaining ¼ teaspoon salt in food processor or blender; blend until smooth.

4. Remove beef to large cutting board; shred with two forks. Combine shredded meat with 1 cup cooking liquid. Discard remaining cooking liquid. Serve on tortillas with sauce. Top as desired.

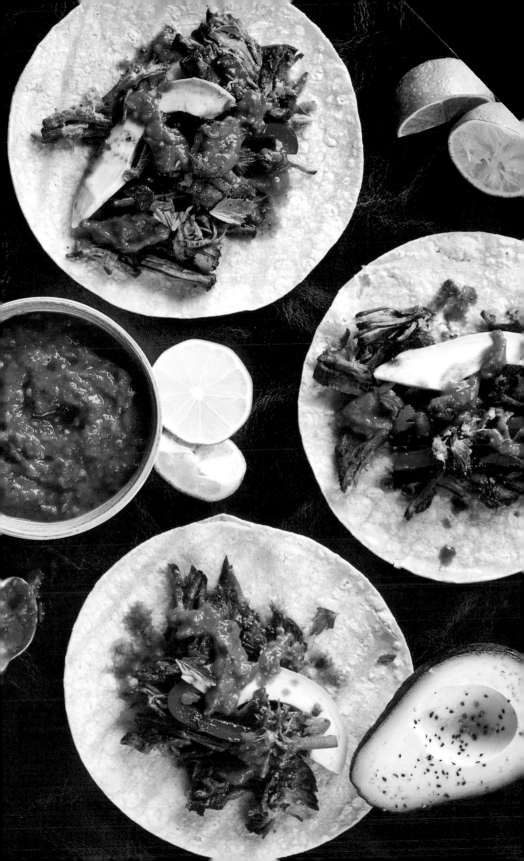

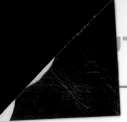

SOUTHWESTERN FLATBREAD WITH BLACK BEANS AND CORN

MAKES 4 SERVINGS

¼ cup prepared green chile enchilada sauce

2 oval flatbreads, each about 7½×11 inches

2 cups (8 ounces) shredded Monterey Jack cheese

1 can (about 14 ounces) black beans, rinsed and drained

1 cup frozen corn, thawed

½ cup finely diced red onion

½ teaspoon kosher salt

1 teaspoon olive oil

2 tablespoons chopped fresh cilantro

1 avocado, diced

Lime wedges (optional)

1. Preheat oven to 425°F. Place wire rack on top of baking sheet.

2. Spread enchilada sauce evenly on top of each flatbread, sprinkle evenly with cheese. Combine beans, corn, onion, salt and oil in medium bowl. Layer mixture on top of cheese. Place flatbreads on rack on baking sheet. Bake 12 minutes or until flatbread is golden and crisp, and cheese is melted. Remove from oven. Sprinkle with cilantro and avocado.

3. Cut each flatbread crosswise into 4 pieces. Serve with lime wedges, if desired.

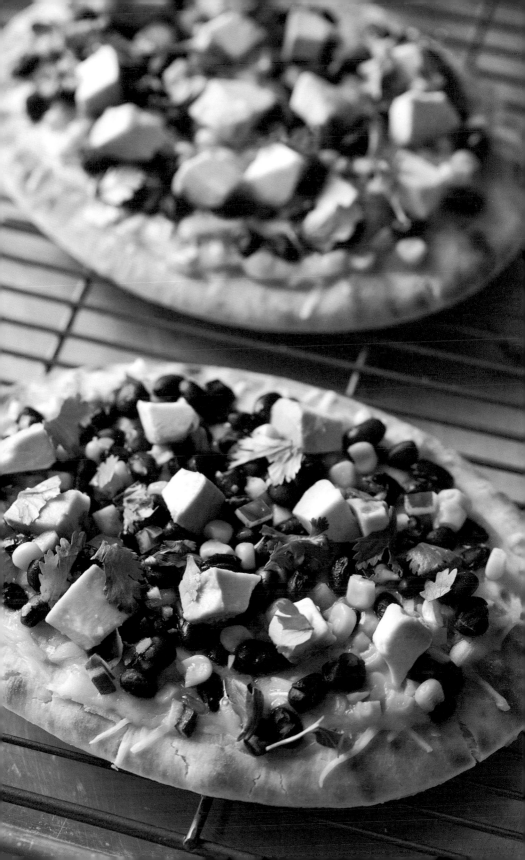

SALSA BACON BURGERS WITH GUACAMOLE

MAKES 4 BURGERS

1 **pound ground beef**

1 **packet (1.25 ounces) ORTEGA® Taco Seasoning Mix**

¼ **cup ORTEGA® Salsa, any variety**

2 **ripe avocados**

1 **packet (1 ounce) ORTEGA® Guacamole Seasoning Mix**

4 **hamburger buns**

8 **slices cooked bacon**

COMBINE ground beef, taco seasoning mix and salsa in large mixing bowl. With clean hands, form meat mixture into 4 patties.

CUT avocados in half and remove pits. Scoop out avocado meat and smash in small bowl. Add guacamole seasoning mix. Set aside.

HEAT large skillet over medium heat; cook burgers 5 minutes. Flip burgers and continue to cook another 7 minutes.

PLACE burgers on bottom of buns. Top each burger with 2 slices bacon, dollop of guacamole and top bun.

PREP TIME: 10 minutes
START TO FINISH: 25 minutes

TIP   Make burgers half the size to create great sliders.

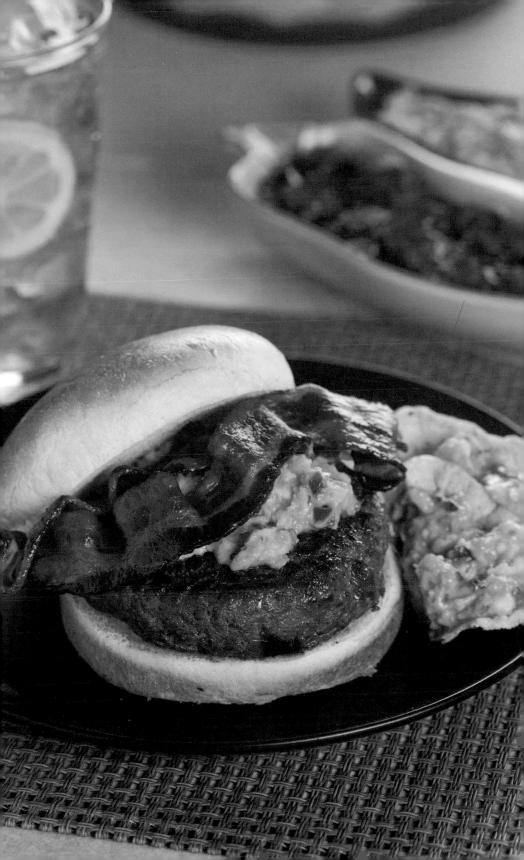

SOUTHWESTERN SCALLOPS

1 pound bay scallops or 1 pound sea scallops, cut into quarters

½ cup lime juice

⅓ cup olive oil

1 teaspoon grated lime peel

1 green onion with top, sliced diagonally into ½-inch pieces

2 tablespoons chopped fresh cilantro

1 tablespoon chopped fresh parsley

Salt

Black pepper

½ cup Italian-style roasted peppers, cut into thin strips

1 avocado

Lime juice

1 medium tomato, coarsely chopped

1 medium tomato, thinly sliced and slices cut into halves

1. Bring 3 inches salted water in large saucepan over high heat to a boil. Reduce heat to low. Add scallops; poach 1 minute. Immediately drain and rinse with cold water.

2. Whisk ½ cup lime juice, oil and lime peel in medium bowl until combined. Stir in scallops, green onion, cilantro and parsley. Season to taste with salt and black pepper. Stir in roasted peppers. Refrigerate, covered, 1 hour or until chilled.

3. To serve, slice avocado; toss with lime juice. Add avocado and chopped tomato to scallop mixture. Spoon into serving plate. Arrange tomato slices around edge of plate.

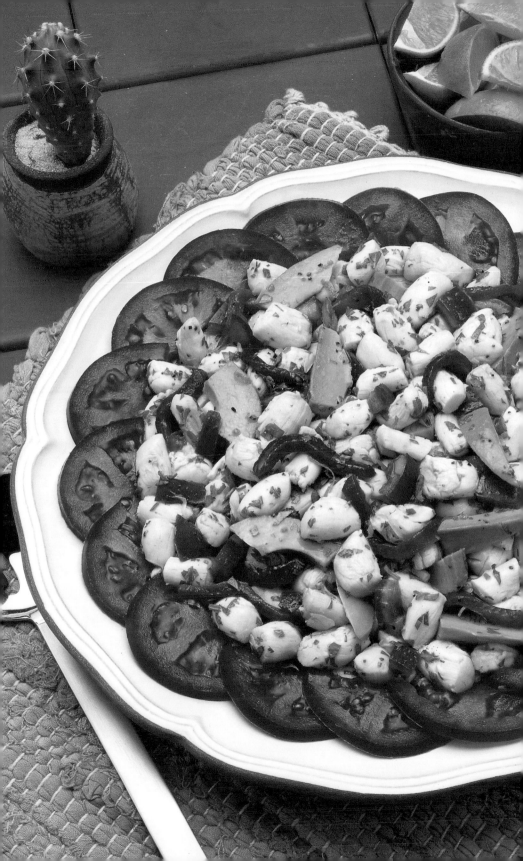

SOFT TACOS WITH CHICKEN

MAKES 8 TACOS

8 (6- or 7-inch) corn tortillas

2 tablespoons butter or margarine

1 medium onion, chopped

1½ cups shredded cooked chicken

1 can (4 ounces) diced mild green chiles, drained

2 tablespoons chopped fresh cilantro

1 cup (½ pint) sour cream

Salt

Black pepper

1½ cups (6 ounces) shredded Monterey Jack cheese

1 large avocado, sliced

Green taco sauce

1. Stack and wrap tortillas in foil. Warm in 350°F oven 15 minutes or until heated through.

2. Melt butter in large skillet over medium heat. Add onion; cook until tender. Add chicken, green chiles and cilantro. Cook 3 minutes or until mixture is hot. Reduce heat to low. Stir in sour cream; season with salt and pepper. Heat gently; do not boil.

3. To assemble tacos, spoon about 3 tablespoons chicken mixture into center of each tortilla; sprinkle with 2 tablespoons cheese. Top with avocado; drizzle with 1 to 2 teaspoons taco sauce. Sprinkle tacos with remaining cheese. Roll tortilla into cone shape or fold in half to eat.

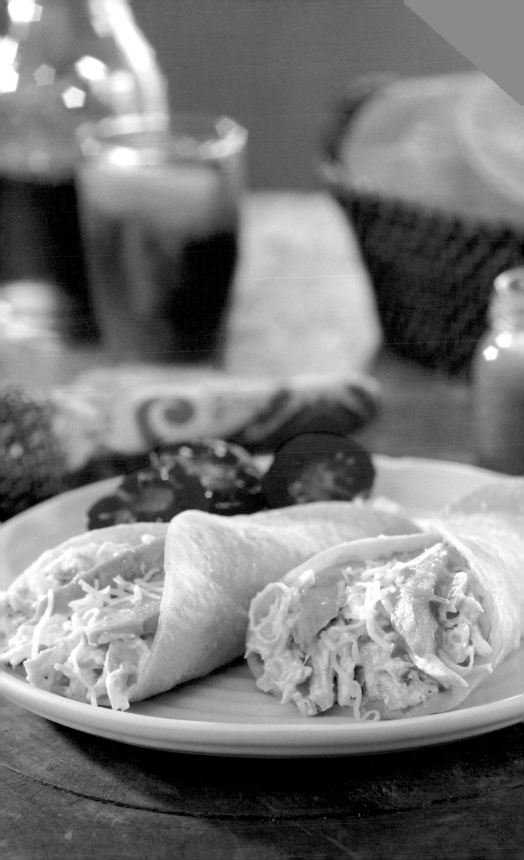

-SEARED HALIBUT STEAKS WITH AVOCADO SALSA

MAKES 4 SERVINGS

4 tablespoons chipotle salsa, divided

½ teaspoon salt, divided

4 small (4 to 5 ounces) *or* 2 large (8 to 10 ounces) halibut steaks, cut ¾ inch thick

½ cup diced tomato

½ ripe avocado, diced

2 tablespoons chopped cilantro (optional)

Lime wedges (optional)

1. Combine 2 tablespoons salsa and ¼ teaspoon salt in small bowl; spread over both sides of halibut.

2. Heat large nonstick skillet over medium heat until hot. Add halibut; cook 4 to 5 minutes per side or until fish is opaque in center.

3. Meanwhile, combine remaining 2 tablespoons salsa, ¼ teaspoon salt, tomato, avocado and cilantro, if desired, in small bowl. Mix well and spoon over cooked fish. Garnish with lime wedges.

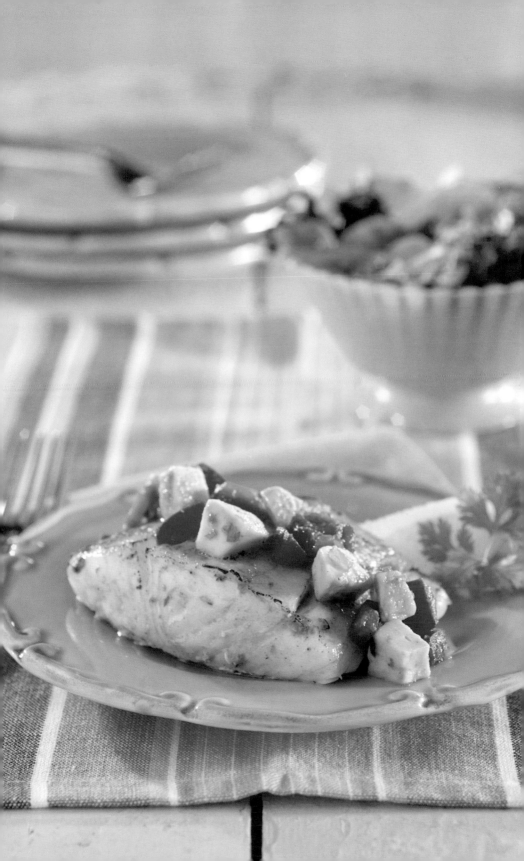

SLOW COOKER GREEN CHILE PULLED PORK SANDWICHES

MAKES 8 SERVINGS

3½ to 4 pounds pork shoulder

1 teaspoon salt

½ teaspoon black pepper

1 can (about 14 ounces) diced tomatoes with mild green chiles, undrained

1 cup chopped onion

½ cup water

2 tablespoons fresh lime juice

1 teaspoon ground cumin

1 teaspoon minced garlic

2 whole canned chipotle peppers in adobo sauce, minced

8 hard rolls or hoagie buns

½ cup sour cream

2 ripe avocados, sliced

3 tablespoons chopped fresh cilantro (optional)

SLOW COOKER DIRECTIONS

1. Season pork with salt and black pepper and place in slow cooker.

2. Combine tomatoes, onion, water, lime juice, cumin, garlic and chipotle peppers in medium bowl. Pour over pork. Cover and cook on LOW 7 to 8 hours or until pork shreds easily when poked with fork or spoon.

3. Remove pork to cutting board and cool slightly. Remove any fat from surface of meat and discard. Shred pork with two forks. Return pork to cooking liquid; stir to combine. Serve on rolls, topping each sandwich with about 1 tablespoon sour cream, avocado slices and a pinch of chopped cilantro, if desired.

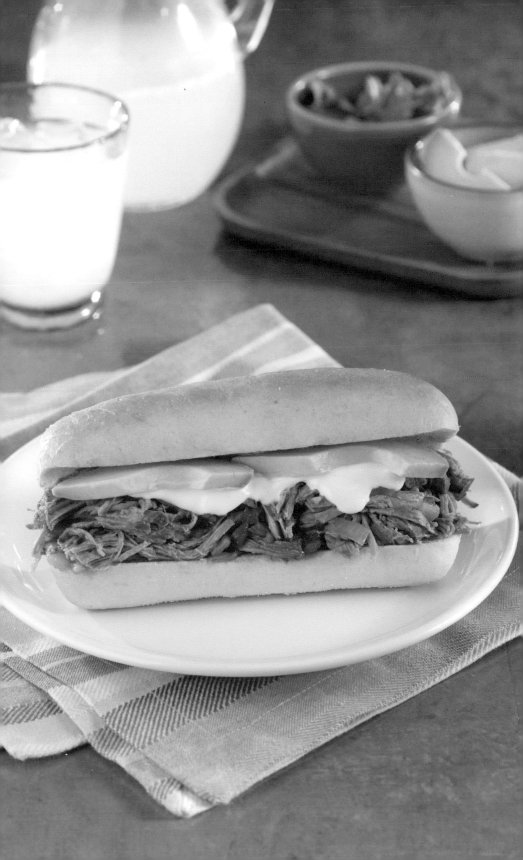

PIZZA MEXICANA

2 tablespoons olive oil

1 medium red onion, diced

1 can (14½ ounces) diced tomatoes, drained

1 can (4 ounces) chopped green chilies, drained

¼ cup chopped fresh cilantro, divided

1 can (16 ounces) refried beans

4 (4 ounces each) prepared Italian bread shells

2 cups (8 ounces) SARGENTO® Fine Cut Shredded 4 Cheese Mexican

Sour cream, sliced ripe avocado (optional)

1. Heat oil in large skillet over medium heat. Add onion; cook 5 minutes, stirring occasionally. Add tomatoes and chilies; cook 5 minutes or until most of liquid evaporates, stirring occasionally. Stir in 2 tablespoons cilantro.

2. Spread beans evenly over bread shells; top with tomato mixture and sprinkle with cheese. Place on large baking sheet.

3. Bake in preheated 450°F oven 10 to 12 minutes or until cheese is melted and crust is browned and crisp. Cut each bread shell into wedges; sprinkle with remaining cilantro. Garnish with sour cream and avocado, if desired.

PREP TIME: 20 minutes
COOK TIME: 18 minutes

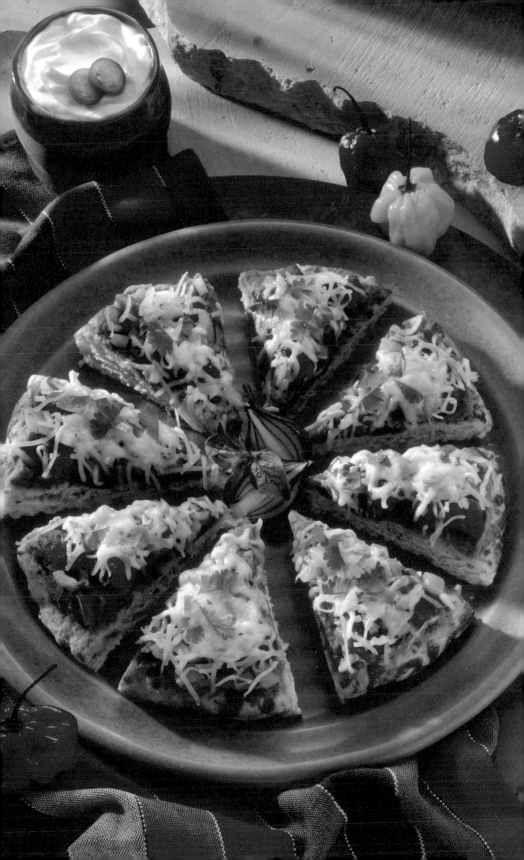

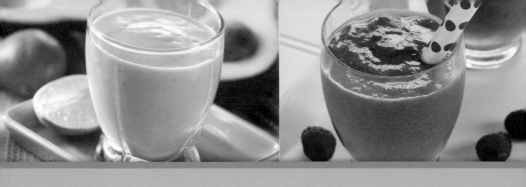

DESSERTS & SMOOTHIES

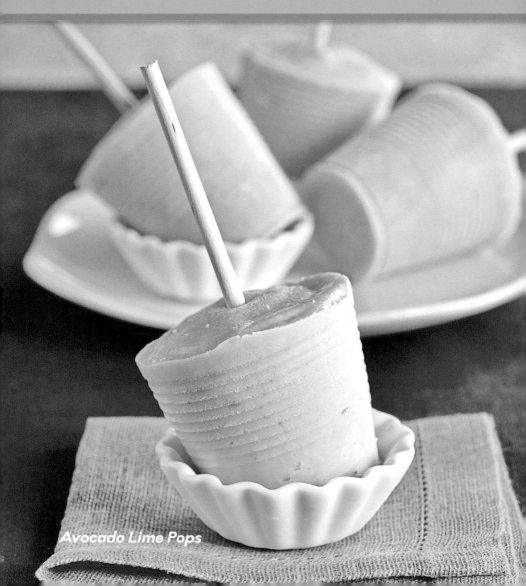

Avocado Lime Pops

AVOCADO LIME POPS

MAKES 6 POPS

1 avocado

1 cup sugar

   Juice and grated peel of
    2 limes

1 cup milk

¼ teaspoon vanilla

6 (5-ounce) plastic cups or
   paper cups or pop molds

6 pop sticks

1. Combine avocado, sugar, lime juice, lime peel, milk and vanilla in blender or food processor; blend until smooth.

2. Pour mixture into cups. Cover top of each cup with small piece of foil. Freeze 1 hour.

3. Insert sticks through center of foil. Freeze 4 hours or until firm.

4. To serve, remove foil and gently twist frozen pops out of plastic cups or peel away paper cups.

VARIATION: **Make these plain pops more appealing by using plastic cups, which give the pops a ridged texture.**

AVOCADO ICE CREAM

MAKES ABOUT 1¹/₂ QUARTS

4 cups milk
1 cup sugar, divided
1 vanilla bean*
2 whole eggs
1 egg yolk

3 ripe avocados
¼ cup fresh lime juice

Or, substitute 1½ teaspoons vanilla for vanilla bean. Add to milk in step 1. Omit step 2.

1. Combine milk, ¾ cup sugar and vanilla bean in medium saucepan. Cook and stir over medium-high heat just until milk begins to boil; remove from heat.

2. Cut vanilla bean in half lengthwise. Scrape seeds into saucepan; add bean halves to saucepan.

3. Combine remaining ¼ cup sugar, whole eggs and egg yolk in large bowl. Beat mixture until frothy and light lemon color. Continue whisking mixture while very slowly pouring in 1 cup hot milk mixture.

4. Slowly pour egg mixture into saucepan with vanilla bean. Cook over medium heat and whisk slowly until first bubble forms. *Do not boil.*

5. Pour custard mixture through fine-meshed sieve into medium bowl set in ice water; stir custard mixture until cool. Cover and refrigerate about 1 hour or until cold.

6. Combine avocados and lime juice in medium bowl. Mash with wooden spoon or potato masher. Press avocado mixture through fine-meshed strainer with rubber spatula; stir into custard mixture.

7. Freeze in ice cream maker according to manufacturer's directions.

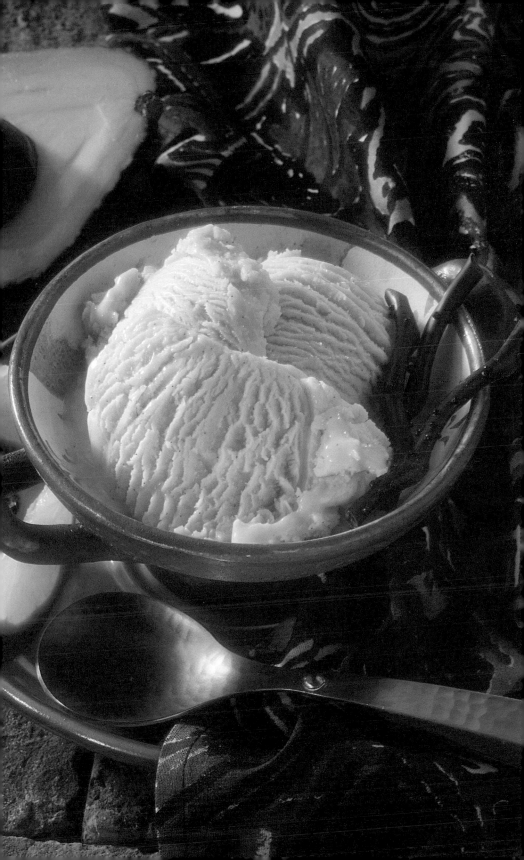

TROPICAL AVOCADO SMOOTHIE

MAKES 4 TO 5 SERVINGS

Pulp of 1 medium avocado

2 cans (12 fluid ounces *each*) NESTLÉ® CARNATION® Evaporated Lowfat 2% Milk, *chilled**

¼ cup granulated sugar or to taste

1 teaspoon grated lime peel (optional)

Crushed ice (optional)

*May use 2 cans (12 fluid ounces each) CARNATION® Evaporated Fat Free Milk.

PLACE avocado, evaporated milk, sugar and lime peel in blender container; cover. Blend for 30 to 45 seconds until smooth.

SERVE in glasses. Top with crushed ice, if desired.

PREP TIME: 5 minutes

NOTE: If a thinner drink is desired, blend in 1 cup ice cubes with drink ingredients.

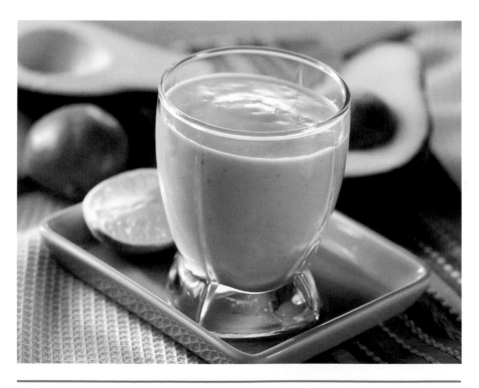

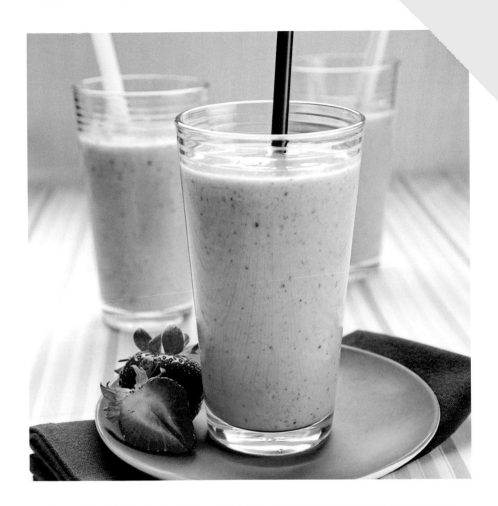

CREAMY STRAWBERRY-BANANA SHAKE

MAKES 2 SERVINGS

1½ **cups ice cubes**

½ **banana**

½ **cup fresh strawberries, hulled**

½ **cup orange juice beverage**

¼ **avocado**

1. Combine ice, banana, strawberries, orange juice beverage and avocado in blender; blend until smooth.

2. Pour into two glasses.

DAIRY-FREE RASPBERRY SMOOTHIE

MAKES 2 SERVINGS

1 cup almond milk

2 cups frozen raspberries

½ avocado

2 tablespoons lemon juice

Combine almond milk, raspberries, avocado and lemon juice in blender; blend until smooth. Serve immediately.

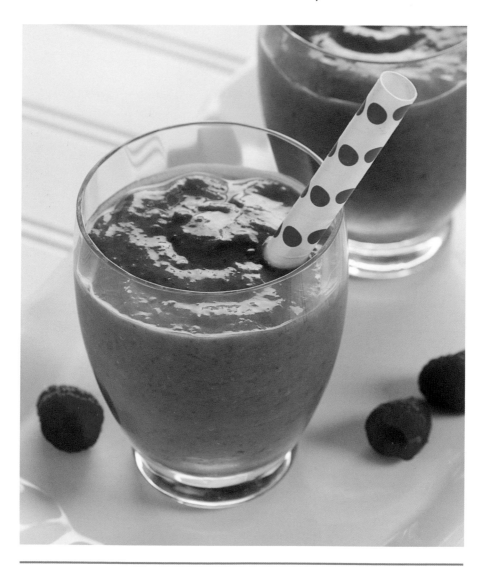

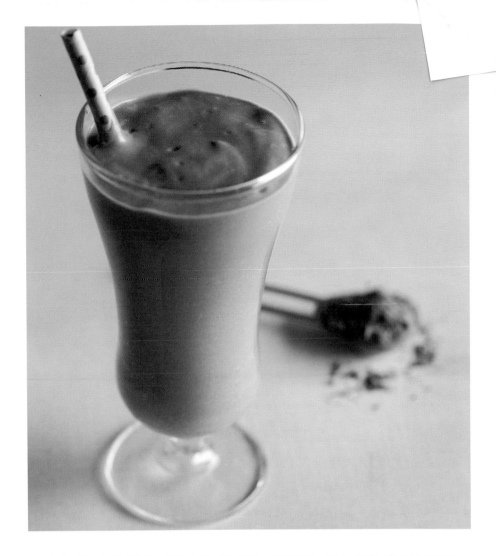

CREAMY CHOCOLATE SMOOTHIE

MAKES 1 SERVING

1 cup unsweetened almond milk

1 frozen banana

½ avocado

1 tablespoon unsweetened cocoa powder

1 tablespoon honey

Combine almond milk, banana, avocado, cocoa and honey in blender; blend until smooth. Serve immediately.

TRIPLE GREEN SMOOTHIE

MAKES 2 SERVINGS

2 cups seedless green grapes   **½ avocado**
1 kiwi, peeled and quartered

Combine grapes, kiwi and avocado in blender; blend until smooth. Serve immediately.

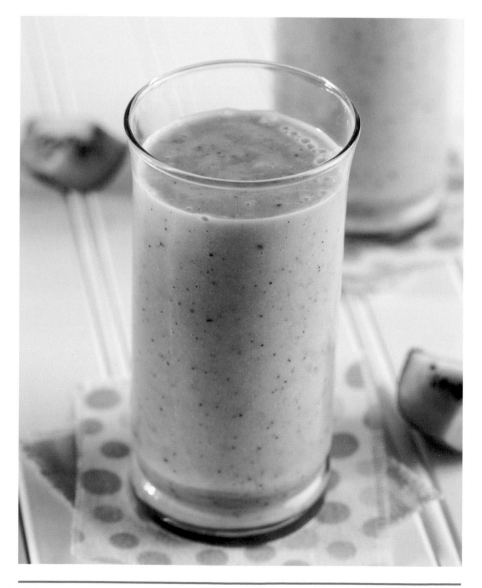

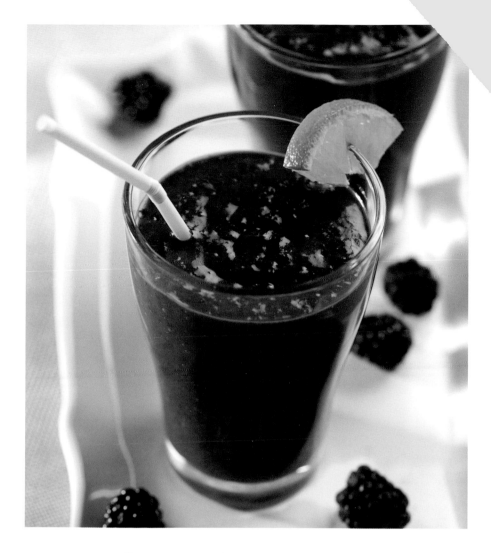

SUPER C SMOOTHIE

MAKES 3 SERVINGS

⅔ cup water

2 navel oranges, peeled and seeded

2 cups frozen blackberries

2 cups baby kale

1 avocado

2 tablespoons honey

Combine water, oranges, blackberries, kale, avocado and honey in blender; blend until smooth. Serve immediately.

AR-AVOCADO SMOOTHIE

MAKES 2 SERVINGS

1½ **cups ice cubes**
 1 **pear, peeled and cubed**
 1 **cup apple juice**
½ **avocado**

½ **cup fresh mint**
 2 **tablespoons fresh lime juice**

1. Combine ice, pear, apple juice, avocado, mint and lime juice in blender; blend until smooth.

2. Pour into two glasses.

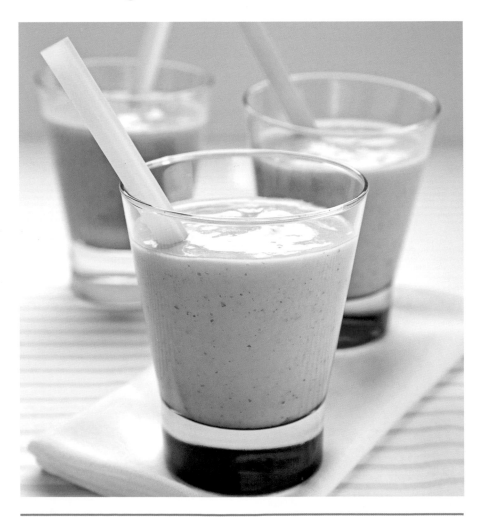

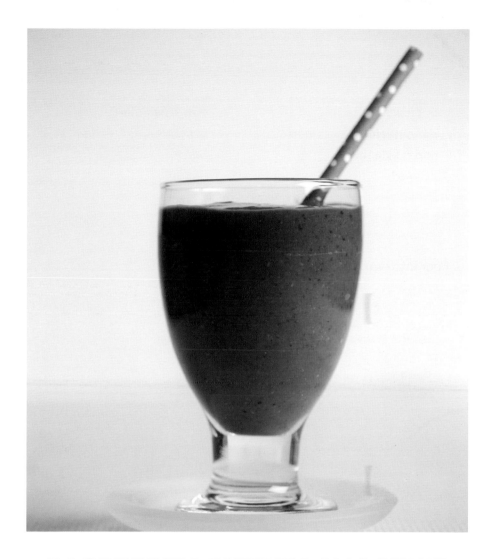

RASPBERRY CHERRY SMOOTHIE

MAKES 2 SERVINGS

⅔ **cup apple juice**

1 **cup frozen raspberries**

1 **cup frozen dark sweet cherries, slightly thawed**

½ **avocado**

Combine apple juice, raspberries, cherries and avocado in blender; blend until smooth. Serve immediately.

SUPER BLUE SMOOTHIE

MAKES 2 SERVINGS

½ **cup pomegranate juice**
¼ **cup water**
¾ **cup frozen blueberries**

¾ **cup frozen blackberries**
½ **avocado**
2 **teaspoons honey**

Combine pomegranate juice, water, blueberries, blackberries, avocado and honey in blender; blend until smooth.

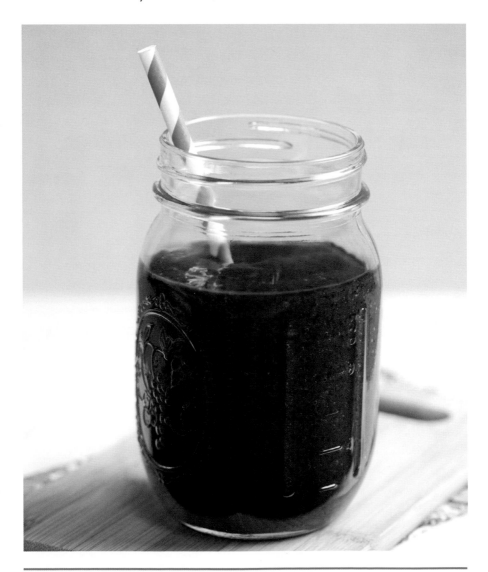

Acknowledgments

The publisher would like to thank the companies listed below for the use of their recipes and/or photographs in this publication.

ConAgra Foods, Inc.

Nestlé USA

Ortega®, A Division of B&G Foods North America, Inc.

Reckitt Benckiser LLC

Sargento® Foods Inc.

Pinnacle Foods

Unilever

METRIC CONVERSION CHART

VOLUME MEASUREMENTS (dry)

$^1/_8$ teaspoon = 0.5 mL
$^1/_4$ teaspoon = 1 mL
$^1/_2$ teaspoon = 2 mL
$^3/_4$ teaspoon = 4 mL
1 teaspoon = 5 mL
1 tablespoon = 15 mL
2 tablespoons = 30 mL
$^1/_4$ cup = 60 mL
$^1/_3$ cup = 75 mL
$^1/_2$ cup = 125 mL
$^2/_3$ cup = 150 mL
$^3/_4$ cup = 175 mL
1 cup = 250 mL
2 cups = 1 pint = 500 mL
3 cups = 750 mL
4 cups = 1 quart = 1 L

VOLUME MEASUREMENTS (fluid)

1 fluid ounce (2 tablespoons) = 30 mL
4 fluid ounces ($^1/_2$ cup) = 125 mL
8 fluid ounces (1 cup) = 250 mL
12 fluid ounces (1$^1/_2$ cups) = 375 mL
16 fluid ounces (2 cups) = 500 mL

WEIGHTS (mass)

$^1/_2$ ounce = 15 g
1 ounce = 30 g
3 ounces = 90 g
4 ounces = 120 g
8 ounces = 225 g
10 ounces = 285 g
12 ounces = 360 g
16 ounces = 1 pound = 450 g

DIMENSIONS

$^1/_{16}$ inch = 2 mm
$^1/_8$ inch = 3 mm
$^1/_4$ inch = 6 mm
$^1/_2$ inch = 1.5 cm
$^3/_4$ inch = 2 cm
1 inch = 2.5 cm

OVEN TEMPERATURES

250°F = 120°C
275°F = 140°C
300°F = 150°C
325°F = 160°C
350°F = 180°C
375°F = 190°C
400°F = 200°C
425°F = 220°C
450°F = 230°C

BAKING PAN SIZES

Utensil	Size in Inches/Quarts	Metric Volume	Size in Centimeters
Baking or	8×8×2	2 L	20×20×5
Cake Pan	9×9×2	2.5 L	23×23×5
(square or	12×8×2	3 L	30×20×5
rectangular)	13×9×2	3.5 L	33×23×5
Loaf Pan	8×4×3	1.5 L	20×10×7
	9×5×3	2 L	23×13×7
Round Layer	8×1½	1.2 L	20×4
Cake Pan	9×1½	1.5 L	23×4
Pie Plate	8×1¼	750 mL	20×3
	9×1¼	1 L	23×3
Baking Dish	1 quart	1 L	—
or Casserole	1½ quart	1.5 L	—
	2 quart	2 L	—